IMAGES OF ENGLAND

THE RADCLIFFE INFIRMARY

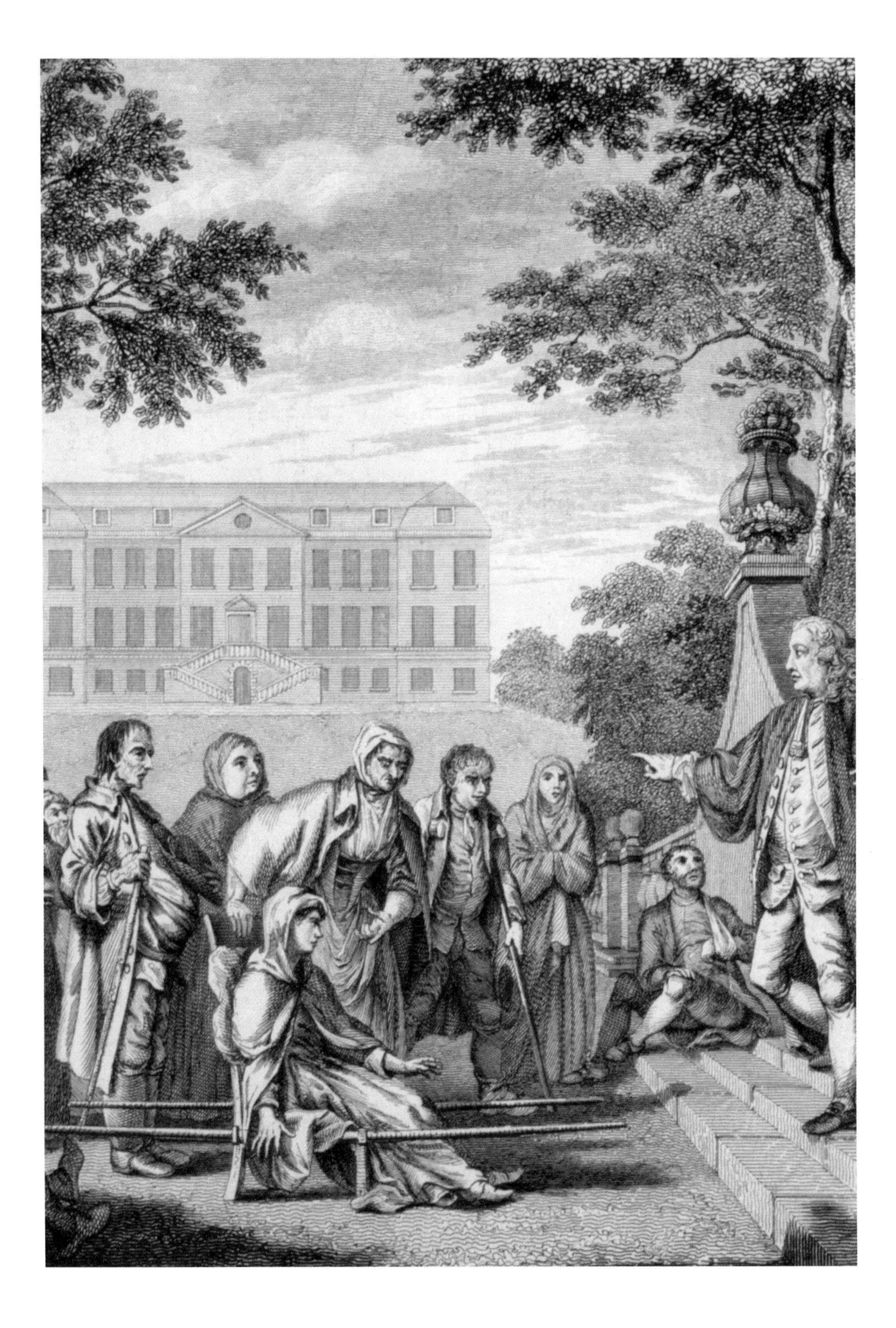

IMAGES OF ENGLAND

THE RADCLIFFE INFIRMARY

ANDREW MOSS

TEMPUS

Frontispiece: John Radcliffe presents his hospital to the poor, sick and lame – an allegorical engraving from the Oxford Almanack in 1760. By this time plans for the hospital had been announced and the engraving would have been used by the trustees to promote the vision and encourage subscribers.

First published 2007

Tempus Publishing Limited
The Mill, Brimscombe Port,
Stroud, Gloucestershire, GL5 2QG
www.tempus-publishing.com

British Library Cataloguing in Publication Data.
A catalogue record for this book is available from the British Library.

ISBN 978 07524 4248 8

Typesetting and origination by Tempus Publishing Limited.
Printed in Great Britain.

Contents

Acknowledgements

The inspiration for this book comes from Oxford Radcliffe Hospitals NHS Trust which has supported the project as one of the ways in which it is marking the closure of a great institution.

In gathering more than 200 images I have tested the patience of many people whose forgiveness I now seek and to whom I owe my thanks. In particular I should like to thank Elizabeth Boardman and Roy Overall of Oxfordshire Health Archives, who started me on my quest and made available their collections. Their guidance has been invaluable.

I was also fortunate to have the support of assistant editor John Chipperfield and librarian Chris McDowell at the *Oxford Mail and Times*. Many of the pictures of the last fifty years come from the *Mail and Times* library and are reproduced with their kind permission.

Jayne Todd, alumni officer, Oxford Medical Alumni, has been exceedingly helpful in making available historic pictures from Oxford Medical School and Peter McKenzie produced fascinating pictures from Oxford Eye Hospital.

Sue Buckingham and members of the Radcliffe Guild of Nurses loaned some of their treasured photographs and I have received valued help from the Cairns library and from past and present staff at the Infirmary including Dorothy Scott, Richard Greenhall, Tim Goodacre, Valerie Thompson, Kathy Gardner and Brenda Spiess. Professor Terence Ryan's detailed knowledge of the hospital has been shared without hesitation as has his collection of photographs. My friends in *Oxford Medical Illustration* have been particularly helpful in copying the most precious items from many sources.

I must also acknowledge my debt to the authors of two books – Alastair Robb-Smith's *A Short History of the Radcliffe Infirmary* and E.J.R. Burrough's *Unity in Diversity*. Robb-Smith in particular brought to life the story of the Infirmary. I have also drawn extensively from early copies of the *Oxford Medical School Gazette*.

I am grateful to Oxford University Press and St Barnabas Church for permission to reproduce the pictures of Thomas and Martha Combe, to Somerville College for the wartime pictures, to Oxfordshire Centre for Local Studies for the use of pictures from their collection and to Oxford Ophthalmological Congress for the picture of Robert Doyne.

Introduction

The closure of the Radcliffe Infirmary brings to an end more than 200 years of service to the community and a proud record of pioneering developments that have marked its name indelibly on the medical map of the world.

This book makes no pretence at being a history of those achievements. That has been done already by historians of far greater experience whose careful research has guided the quest for pictures and informed the wording of captions.

What has been attempted here is to produce a souvenir of a great hospital by using photographs to cast an affectionate backward glance at an establishment whose present and former staff are proud to say 'I trained there' or 'I worked there'.

Almost by definition, it is bound to be incomplete. Where there are no pictures, there is no story. But hopefully enough has been found to make a book which reveals fascinating perspectives on life at the Infirmary in the eighteenth and nineteenth centuries and prompts memories of how things used to be in the not so distant past.

The Radcliffe Infirmary

When John Radcliffe, the highly successful physician, MP and landowner died in 1714, he left a substantial part of his fortune to Oxford and his trustees used it to build the Radcliffe Camera Library, the Infirmary and the Observatory.

The hospital opened in 1770 and was finally completed in 1775 with ninety-four beds on seven wards. By 1875 there were 166 beds on seventeen wards, with 1,300 inpatients, 3,400 outpatients and 1,800 casualties receiving treatment that year.

Oxford Eye Hospital moved to the Infirmary in the late nineteenth century and there were major expansions in the inter-war years, thanks largely to the generosity of William Morris, Lord Nuffield. In 1948, after 178 years of being reliant on charitable donations, the hospital became part of the NHS.

A pioneering hospital

From its earliest days the Infirmary has led the way in advances in medicine, surgery and health care. In the 1770s the surgeon John Grosvenor was one of the first in England to use massage for stiff joints and injured limbs but it was not until 1908 that Dr Walter Turrell was appointed electrotherapeutic physician and revolutionised the practice of physiotherapy through a world-leading department.

Indeed, the early years of the twentieth century were dominated by the appointment of towering figures who established a tradition of pushing the boundaries of medicine and science. After Acland and Osler, Dr Alexander Gibson made ground-breaking discoveries in heart medicine and Dr R.H. Sankey began an X-ray department in a hut in 1907, while E. Cecil Bevers, elected surgeon to the Infirmary in 1915, was among the most able of all the Radcliffe surgeons.

An orthopaedic department led by Arthur Dodds-Parker and Robert Girdlestone was started in 1918 (later the Wingfield Orthopaedic Hospital and now the Nuffield Orthopaedic Centre) and the Infirmary established a department for nervous disorders for the investigation and treatment of patients in the earliest stages of mental disorder, later developed at Littlemore and Warneford hospitals.

At the same time T. Pomfret 'Tommy' Kilner was founding a plastic surgery service which quickly became one of the leading centres in the world and has continued to this day with pioneering surgery through a succession of very able surgeons and productive team work between plastic surgery, neurosurgery and laboratory science.

The idea of an obstetric flying squad, prompted by the number of mothers who were rushed into hospital on the point of death, was pioneered here and its success in saving life and improving care was soon copied elsewhere. The Infirmary was the first in Great Britain to establish an accident service and in 1941, in the most famous of the hospital's clinical 'firsts', the first dose of penicillin was injected into a patient.

The story goes on and in post-war years the hospital has pioneered many developments in medical and nursing practice, including the clinical nursing unit on Beeson ward where nurses took the lead in rehabilitation of elderly patients.

As it ends its life as a hospital, the Infirmary site now starts a new era with Oxford University. Imaginative plans for redevelopment which will retain the handsome eighteenth-century hospital buildings and open views of the neighbouring Observatory are currently being discussed.

Meanwhile the services which have operated for so long in buildings of varying age and suitability, now join Oxford's other outstanding services in new buildings at the John Radcliffe – on the Manor House estate which the Revd George Cronshaw, the then treasurer, persuaded the Infirmary's governors to buy in 1919.

Andrew Moss
January 2007

one

Founders and Benefactors

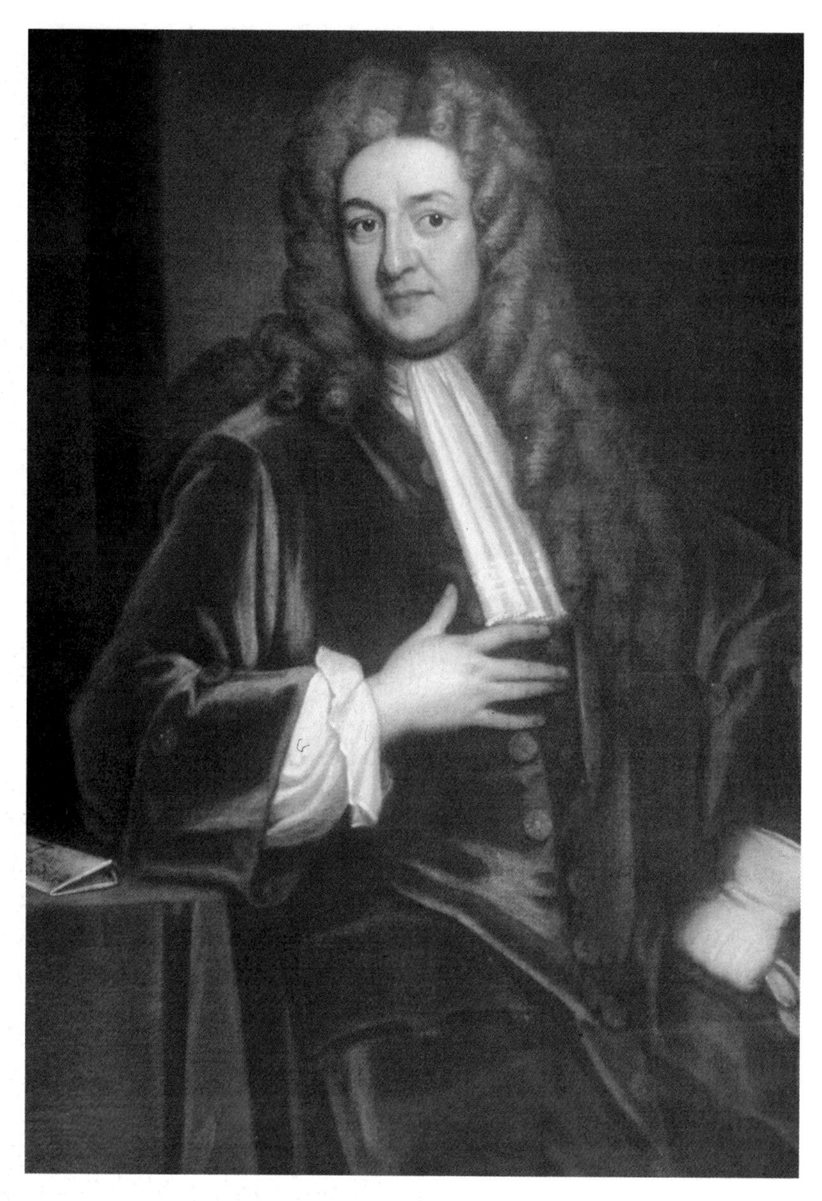

The Radcliffe Infirmary owes its name and its origin to Dr John Radcliffe who came to University College, Oxford from Wakefield in 1665 at the age of thirteen and spent his early years at the university gaining first a BA and then turning to medicine.

He practised in Oxford for a time but in 1684 he went to seek his fortune in London and as well as becoming an immensely successful doctor (he was physician to Mary II, William III and Queen Anne) he was also MP for both Bamber and Buckingham.

His contemporaries described him as forthright, witty and quietly generous, with a caustic and fearless humour which his royal charges were not spared.

He owned two houses in London, a country house at Carshalton and estates in Buckinghamshire, Northamptonshire and Yorkshire, and on his death from apoplexy in 1714 he left £140,000. His trustees used their share of the money to build the Radcliffe Camera Library, the Radcliffe Observatory and the Radcliffe Infirmary.

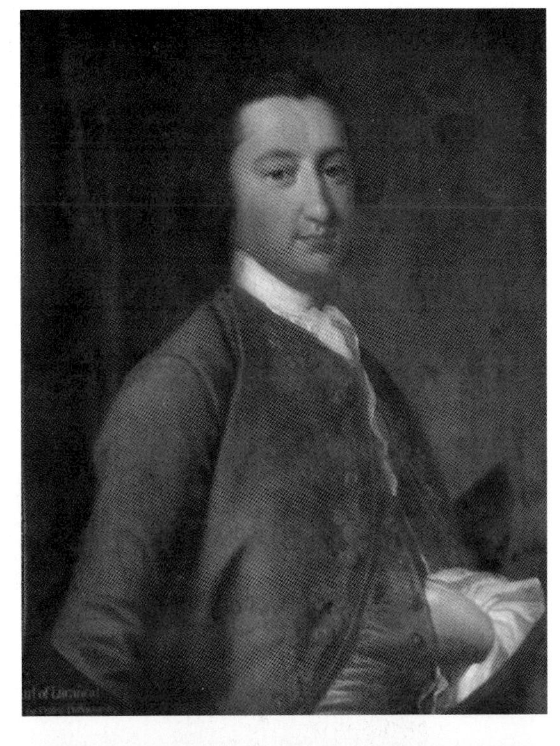

George Henry Lee, third Earl of Lichfield, was one of the trustees of Radcliffe's will and has a reasonable claim to being the driving force in founding the hospital.

He was the first president of the Infirmary, MP for Oxford County, and chancellor of the university in 1762. Described as, 'a jolly and good humoured man, who kept a genial and convivial eye on county, city and university affairs' he successfully drew people of all factions together in support of the hospital. The Oxford antiquary Thomas Walton said of him that he was skilled to lend dignity with ease, to unite affability with propriety and to embellish good sense with all the graces of wit.

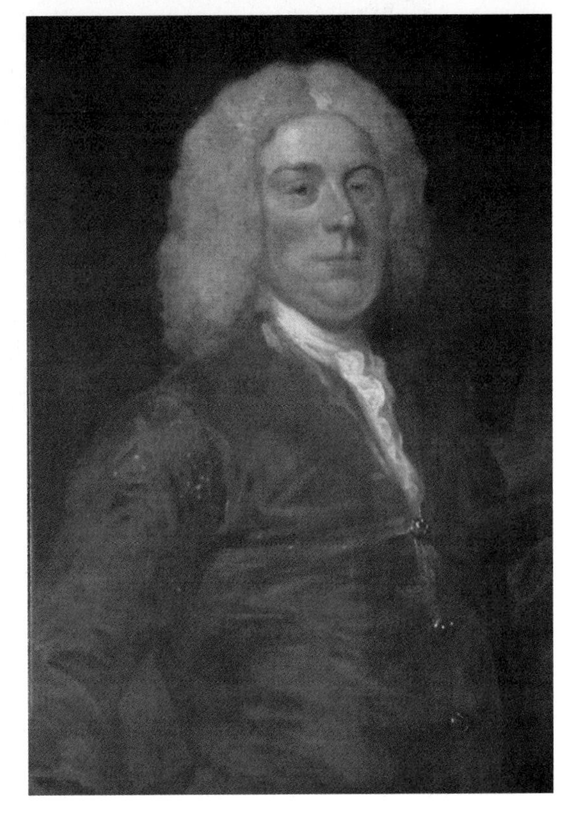

Thomas Rowney 1693-1759
A little round and laughing figure who succeeded his father as MP for the city of Oxford in 1722. He gave Coggins Piece – an area of five and a quarter acres – as the site for the Infirmary and in another act of generosity to the city, paid most of the cost of Oxford Town Hall.

He was a boon companion in politics and pleasure of the Earl of Lichfield in whose company, while out hunting, he was seized with a violent fit of coughing, fell from his horse and died instantly, probably from a stroke.

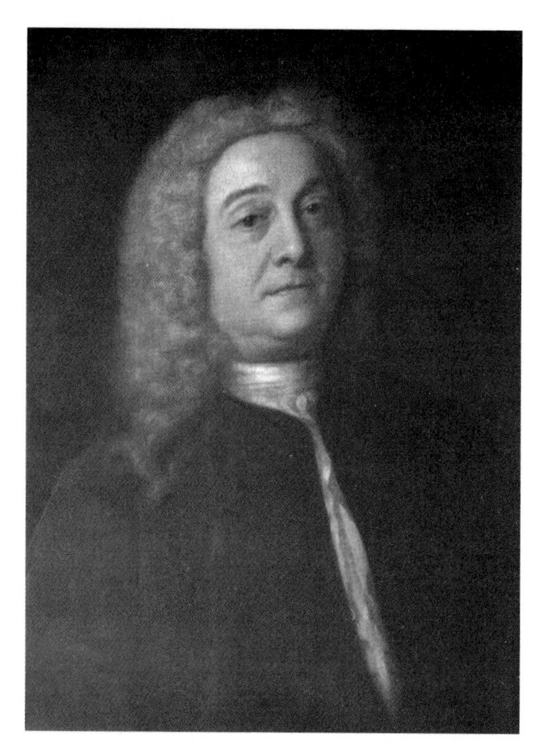

Dr Richard Frewin 1681-1759
A leading Oxford physician, he was one of the first to advocate the need for a hospital, having suffered the loss of three wives and several children. In his will he left £2,000 of which the interest was to be paid, 'to the physician appointed to the new hospital'.

As a result, from 1774 to 1959 a sum of about £60 was shared between the senior physicians, but in 1960 the governors were told it was in breach of NHS regulations and there is now the Frewin Prize for the best memoir submitted by a senior registrar or registrar.

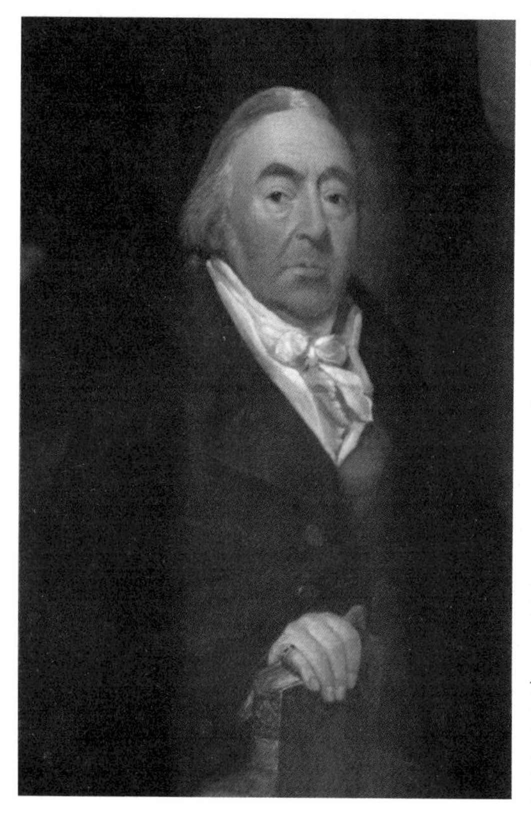

John Grosvenor 1742-1823
One of the four surgeons appointed when the hospital opened in 1770, he stayed on the staff for forty-seven years. He was an excellent surgeon and was one of the first in England to introduce massage to stiff joints and injured limbs. He was noted for his pleasant manners, his hearty address and humorous oddities.

In 1795 he became editor of Jackson's *Oxford Journal*, 'a task which he easily performed during his breakfast hour each morning'. He resigned in 1817 to devote his whole time to the journal, which often reported some of the more remarkable accidents treated at the Infirmary.

Right: Thomas Combe 1796-1872
The chapel was a gift from Thomas Combe, who joined Oxford University Press in 1838 and led its bible printing section into unprecedented prosperity, becoming a rich man in the process.

He was a patron of the arts and collected many Pre-Raphaelite paintings, most of which he left to the university (they are now in the Ashmolean Museum). The chapel was not his only gift to Oxford: he also paid for the Church of St Barnabas in Jericho.

Combe was a governor of the Infirmary and from 1852 to 1872 a member of the committee of management. The chapel was designed by A.W. (later Sir Arthur) Blomfield, and was completed in 1865 at a cost of £3,000. (Oxford University Press)

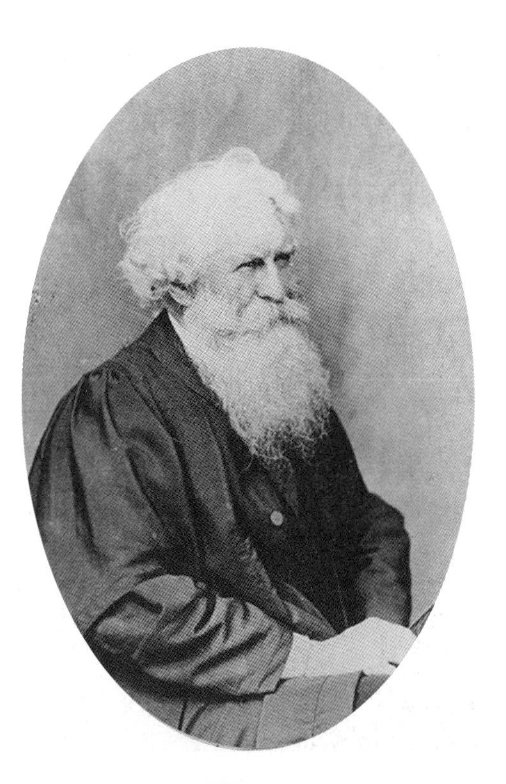

Below: St Luke's Chapel, *c.* 1920. Built in Early English Gothic style, it includes an organ by G.M. Holditch, recognised as an instrument of importance to the national heritage and a lectern carved by the Revd Seymour Ashwell, a member of the committee from 1883 to 1901.

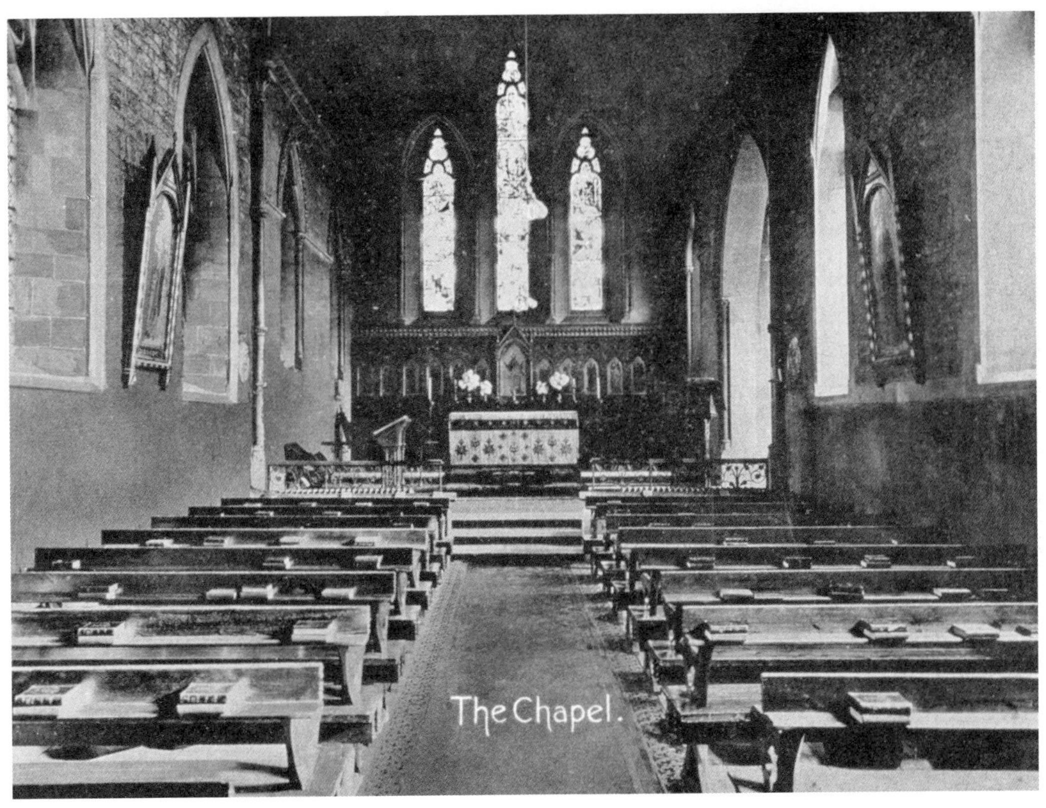

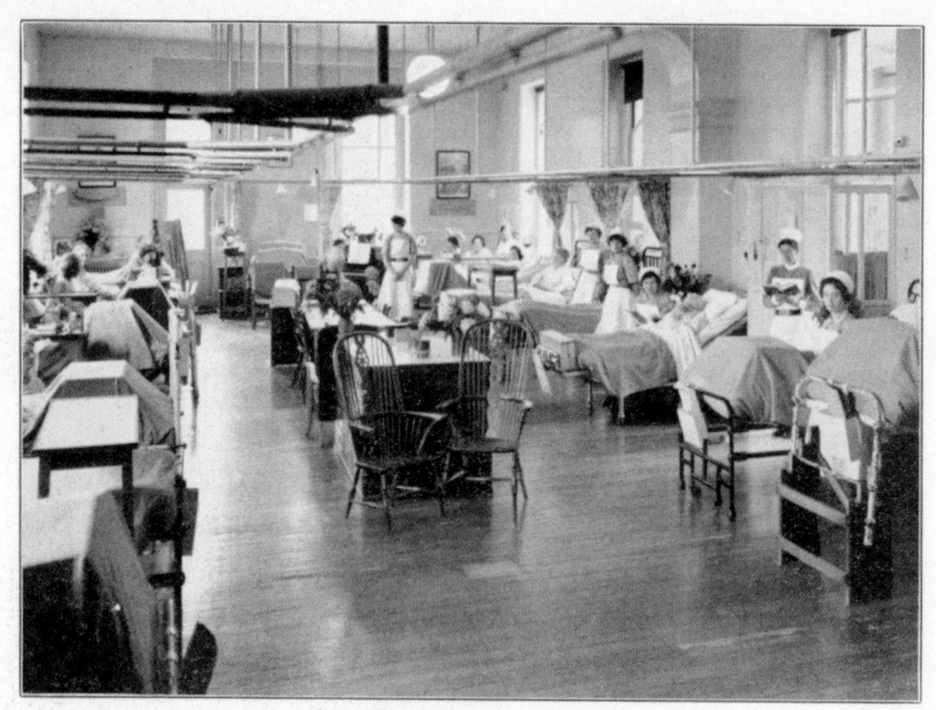

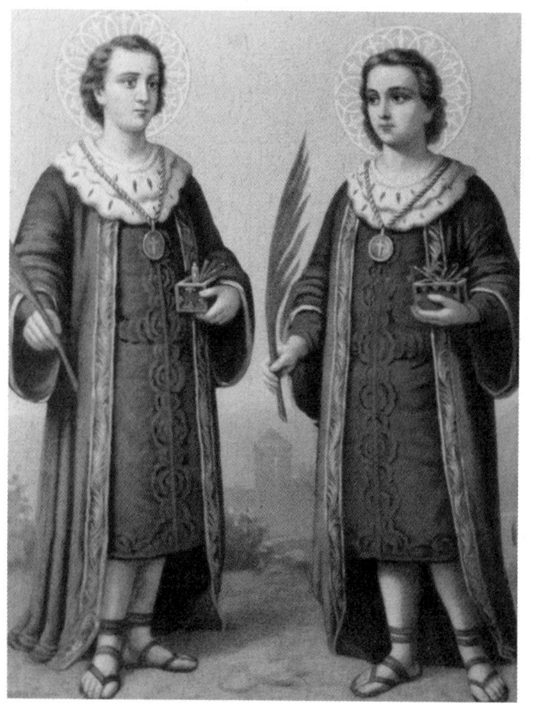

Above: When the chapel opened the custom of an annual sermon and ceremonial procession to the university Church of St Mary's was abandoned, but annual services on St Luke's Day, 18 October, the anniversary of the opening of the hospital, continued for some years. They were often held in St Ebbe's, as this invitation from the 1950s shows. Members of the medical profession (but not the rest of the congregation) were invited to hear a talk on 'Christianity and the everyday life' after the service.

Left: Cosmas and Damian, the patron saints of surgery, were doctors of Arab origin who travelled the world curing the sick and preaching Christianity. They suffered martyrdom in Celicia in the third century AD. This picture of them was sent to the then Matron Agnes Watt, by the Regius Professor Sir William Osler with a note asking for it to be hung in the operations room so that surgeons could seek comfort and inspiration from the saints. It later hung near the chapel.

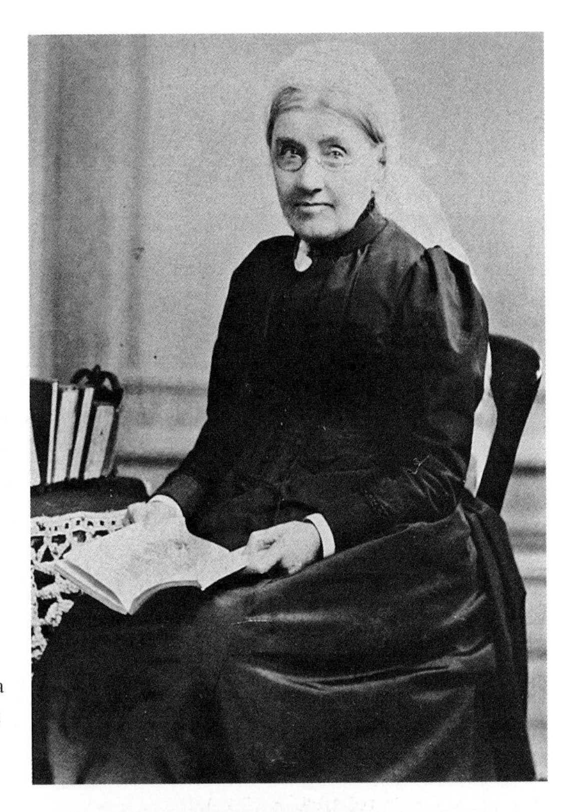

Right: Martha Combe
When the Infirmary opened it only admitted children in emergencies or for major surgery, but in the second half of the nineteenth century the committee began to consider the idea of a children's ward. The first ward, Mordaunt, opened in 1867 but there were outbreaks of diphtheria and then fever and during fumigation in 1874 a fire caused serious damage.

At this point Thomas's widow Martha Combe offered to provide a properly planned children's block, to be designed by Sir Arthur Blomfield. Her offer was accepted with gratitude and the new building was ceremonially opened by Queen Victoria's youngest son, Prince Leopold, in 1877. (St Barnabas Church)

Below: The new children's ward, 1877. It was a white brick building on two floors with eight beds in each ward and its own nurses' room, baths and kitchen. The cost was £2,000.

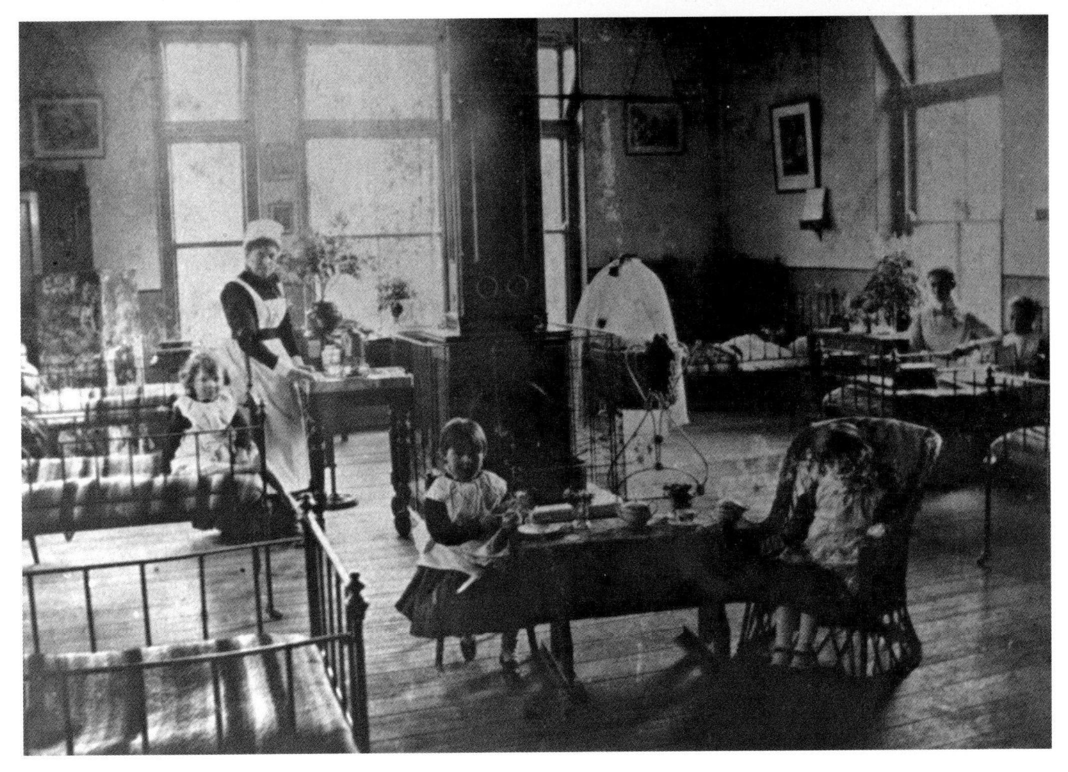

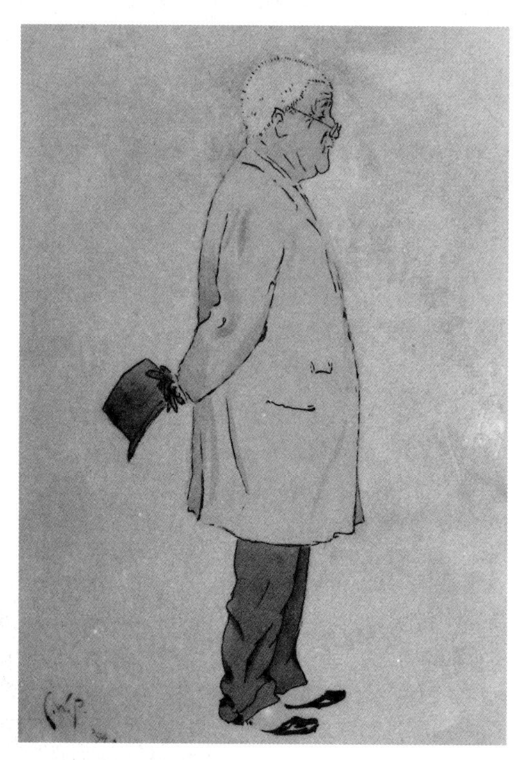

John Briscoe 1820-1908
A surgeon who devoted his whole life to the hospital where he was surgeon apothecary in 1845–57 and honorary surgeon from 1865 until he retired in 1881. He lived in Broad Street and was a regular visitor after retirement. When he died he left his entire fortune of £62,799 to the Infirmary, the largest benefaction in its history (Lord Nuffield's gifts being mostly to the university).

Born in Wales, Briscoe had a practical tact and was kindly in nature. He did all the eye operations as well as general surgery and was described as a careful, but not brilliant operator, immensely practical and a common sense diagnostician who took great care of his patients. The watercolour picture, from 1894, shows him 'observing a case'.

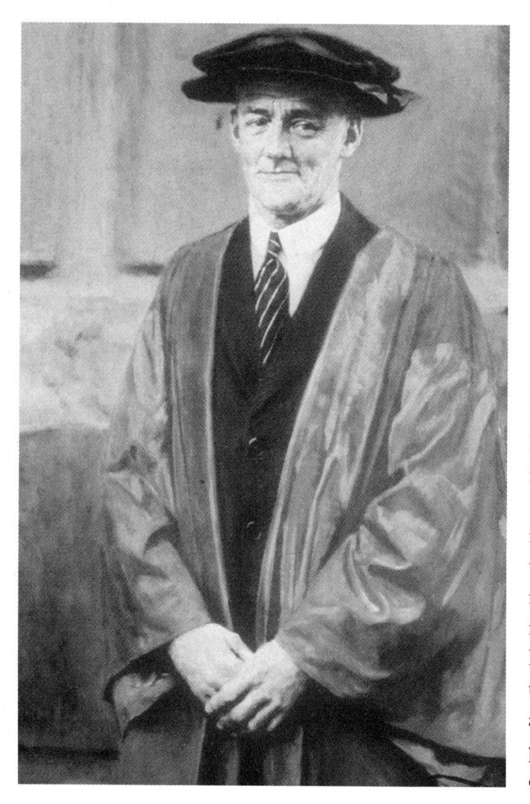

William Morris, Lord Nuffield 1887-1963
Lord Nuffield was a generous benefactor to the hospital and to the university throughout his life. He became vice-president of the Infirmary in 1924 and was president from 1927 until July 1948. In 1928 he provided £38,000 for the maternity home and in 1935 £8,000 for Collier ward. Perhaps most significantly, he provided the money to buy the neighbouring Observatory in 1929 which enabled the expansion of the hospital between the wars. His donations to the university (part of £10 million he gave away in his lifetime) established the Nuffield professorships of surgery, medicine, orthopaedics, obstetrics and anaesthetics in 1937.

two

The Changing Face of the Infirmary

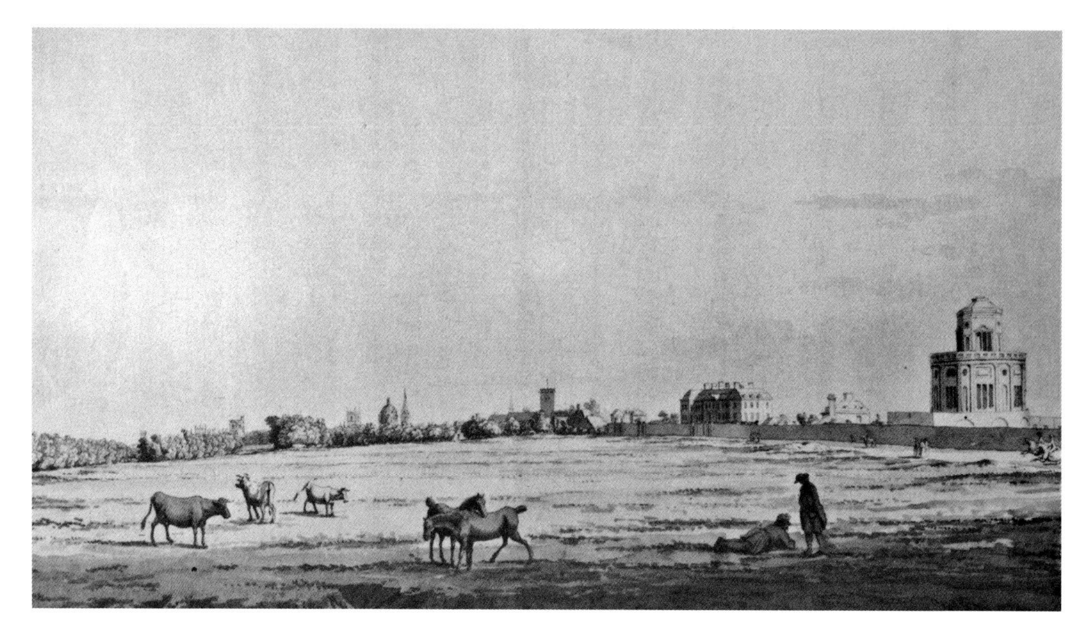

When the Infirmary was built it stood in open fields. This picture from the late eighteenth century shows the three buildings erected by the Radcliffe trustees. The Infirmary in the centre is flanked by the Radcliffe Camera away to the left and the Observatory on the right. Three farms surrounded the hospital and a number of gravel pits were nearby, used by the parish for repairing the roads.

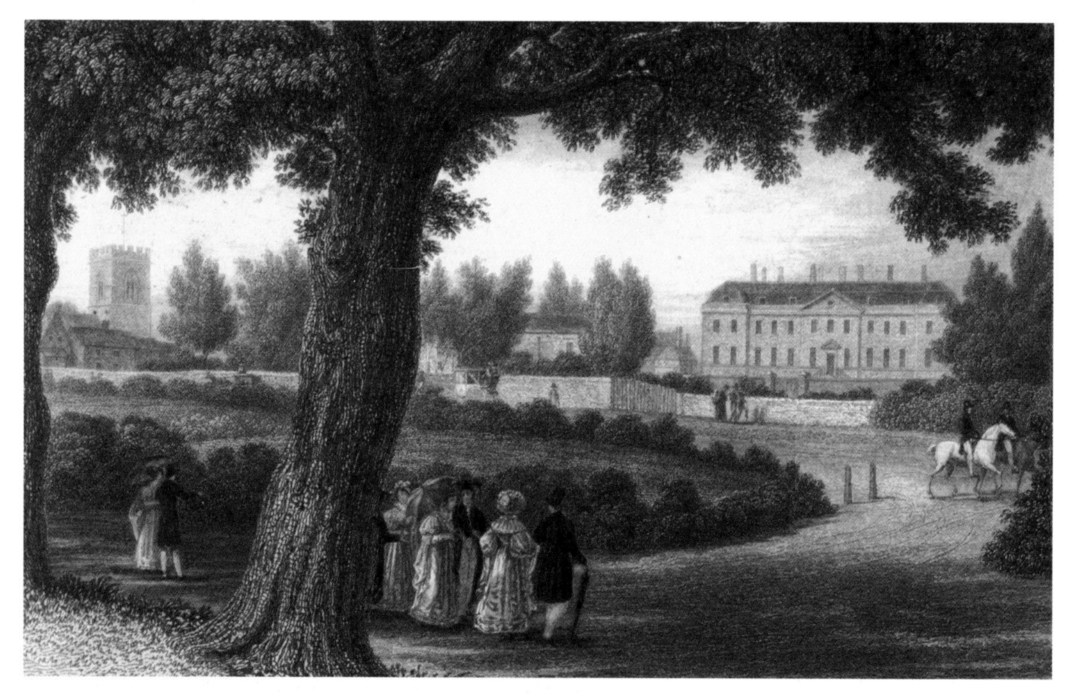

The Infirmary viewed from St Giles. The Royal Oak pub – a popular haunt for generations of staff – would later occupy the site in the foreground. It was in this rural environment that eighteenth-century highwaymen fell upon unsuspecting travellers.

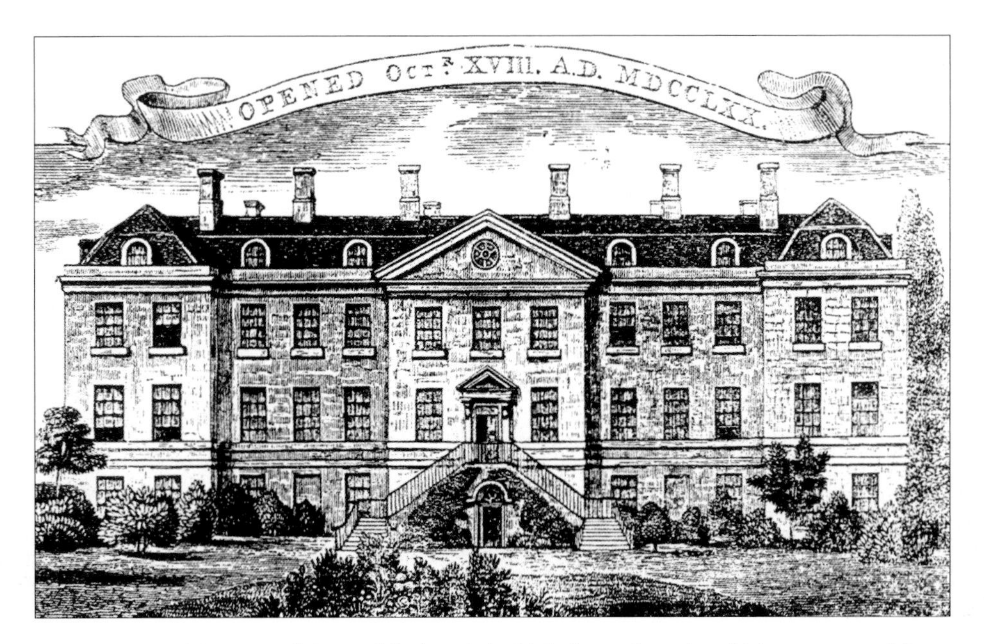

An engraving of the original front of the hospital which shows the stairs which swept gracefully up to the main entrance on the first floor, immediately opposite the board room. This was the route for the governors and the great and the good. Patients and staff entered by the small door at ground level.

The building was designed by Stiff Leadbetter, surveyor to St Paul's Cathedral and architect of Gloucester County Hospital. His plans were presented to the trustees in March 1759 and a contract for £5,692 10*s* signed in the same year. After his death in 1766 the building was completed by John Sanderson of London.

The small, round window provided light for the operating theatre. On the floor below was a small chapel. To either side were the wards. The top floor was staff accommodation.

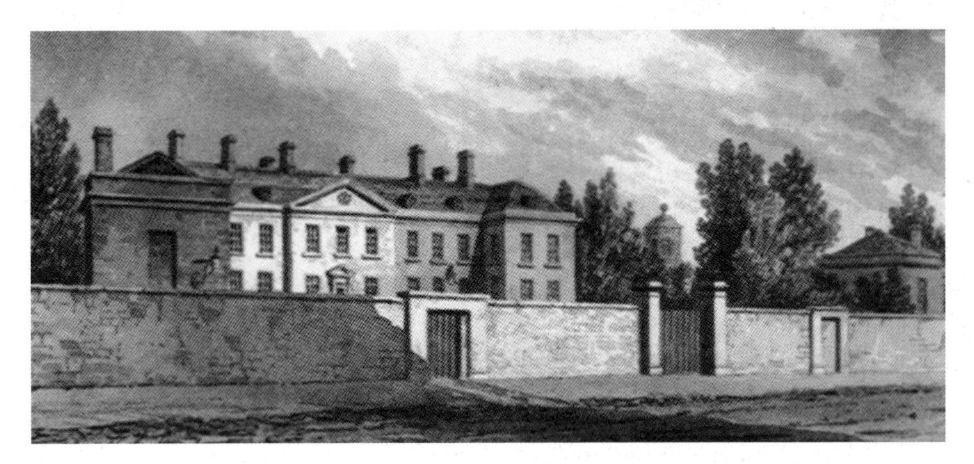

Additions to Leadbetter's original design included a high wall as this engraving by J.C. Buckler in 1821 shows. The wall surrounded the site until 1827 when it was lowered and iron railings erected. The artist, John Buckler, was an architect employed in estate management for Magdalen College who took up a parallel career as an artist during which he made 13,000 drawings providing an invaluable record of churches and public buildings.

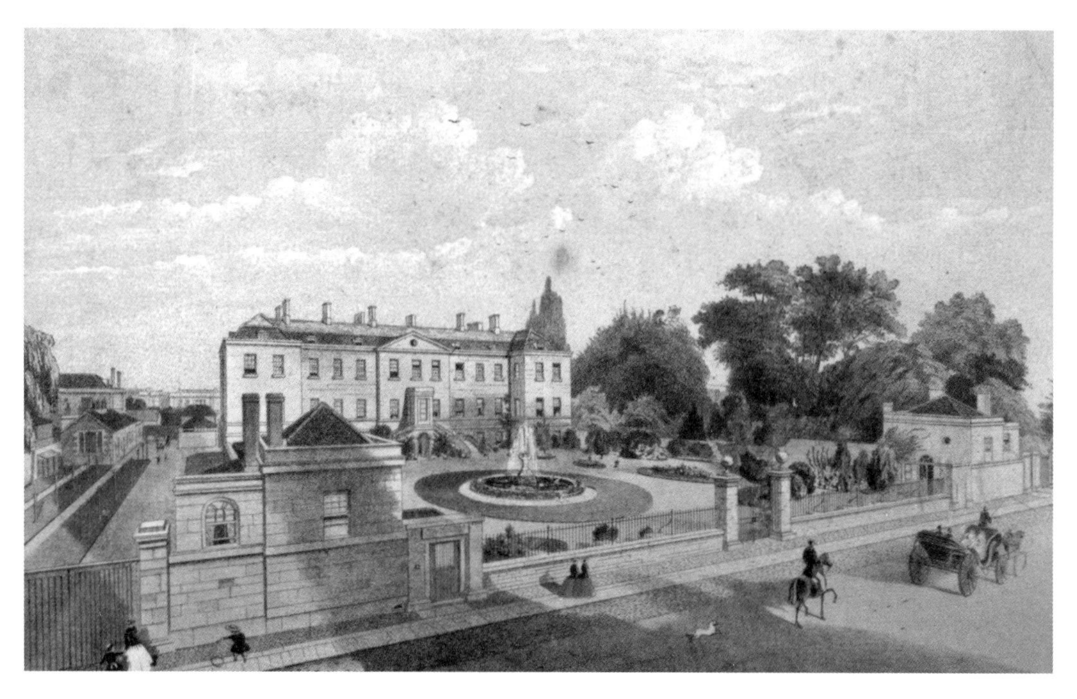

A charming engraving of the hospital with the Triton fountain in place but as yet no chapel on the northern side, *c.* 1860. This would have been produced commercially for sale to the public in the days before photography. For years it hung on the wall of matron's office, but a new matron with new tastes decreed it had to go. Thankfully, it was rescued from a skip by a member of staff and later transferred to the Oxfordshire Health Archives.

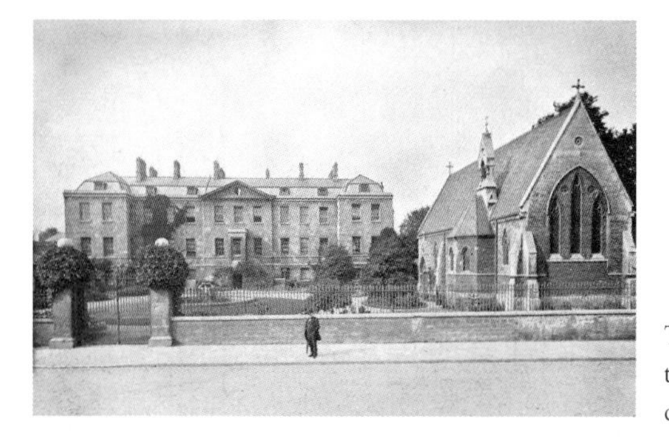

The hospital with St Luke's Chapel on the right and a quizzical passer-by in the centre, *c.* 1890.

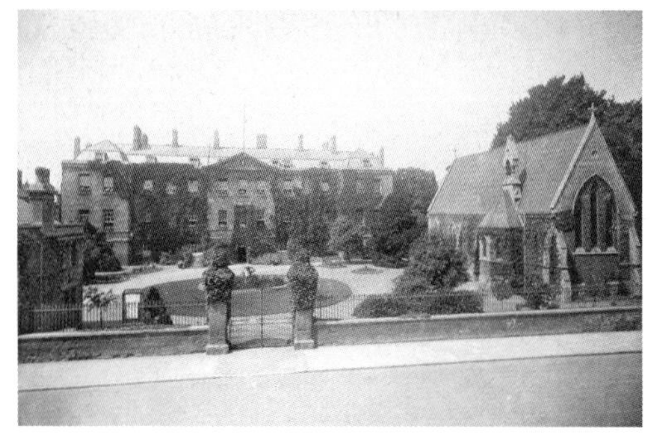

The Infirmary with a luxuriant growth of creeper and ivy over its front and the pillars and railings beside the main gates, *c.* 1900.

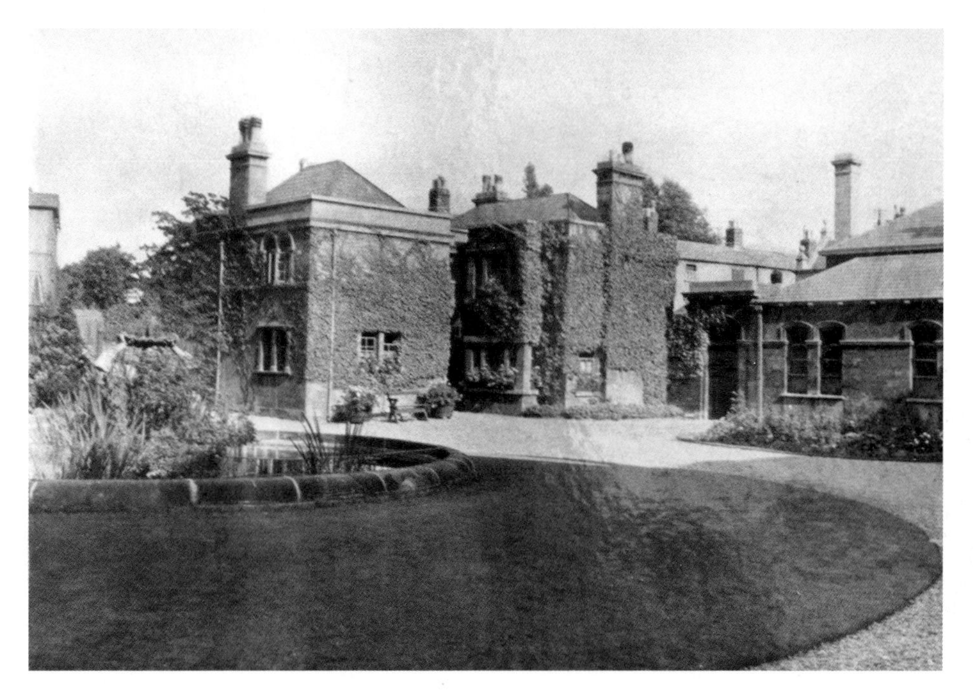

An unusual view across the courtyard, *c.* 1900. The photograph is probably taken from the steps beside the entrance, looking out towards Woodstock Road and St Giles. The buildings shown include the single-storey outpatients (right). They were all demolished to make way for the buildings in the picture below.

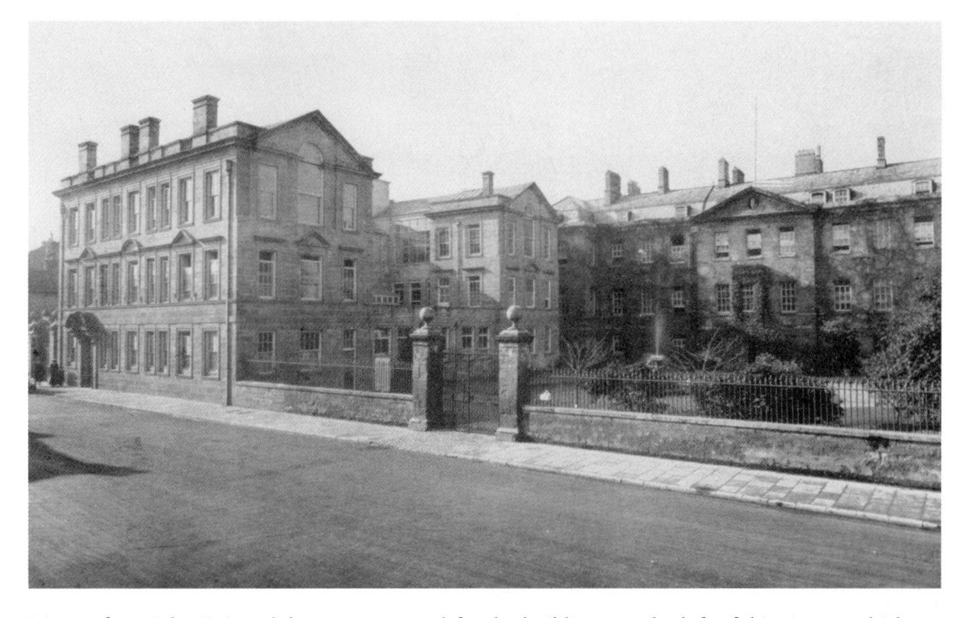

Money from John Briscoe's bequest was used for the buildings on the left of this picture which included a waiting hall and consulting rooms, a casualty operating theatre and a dispensary on the ground floor; electrotherapeutic, X-ray and ear, nose and throat departments on the first floor; and a pathology laboratory, post mortem room and lecture room on the top. They opened in 1913.

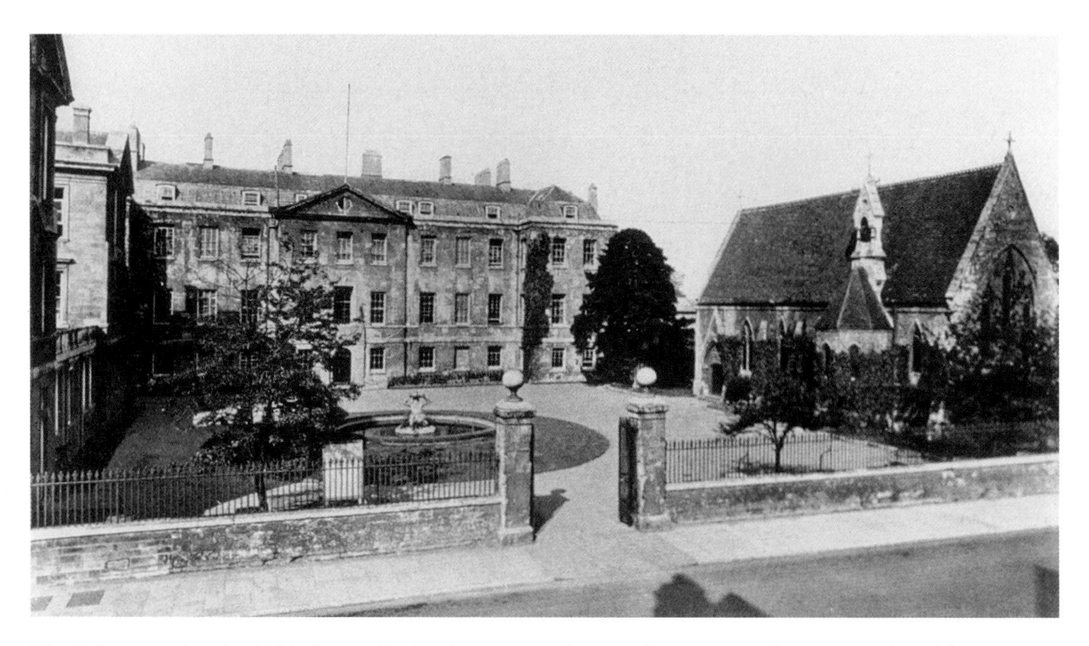

The Infirmary after the 1933 changes by Stanley Hemp. The stairs have gone and a new window fills the space on the first floor, lighting a tall entrance hall. The building retains fine vaulted corridors on the ground and first floors and an original stone staircase.

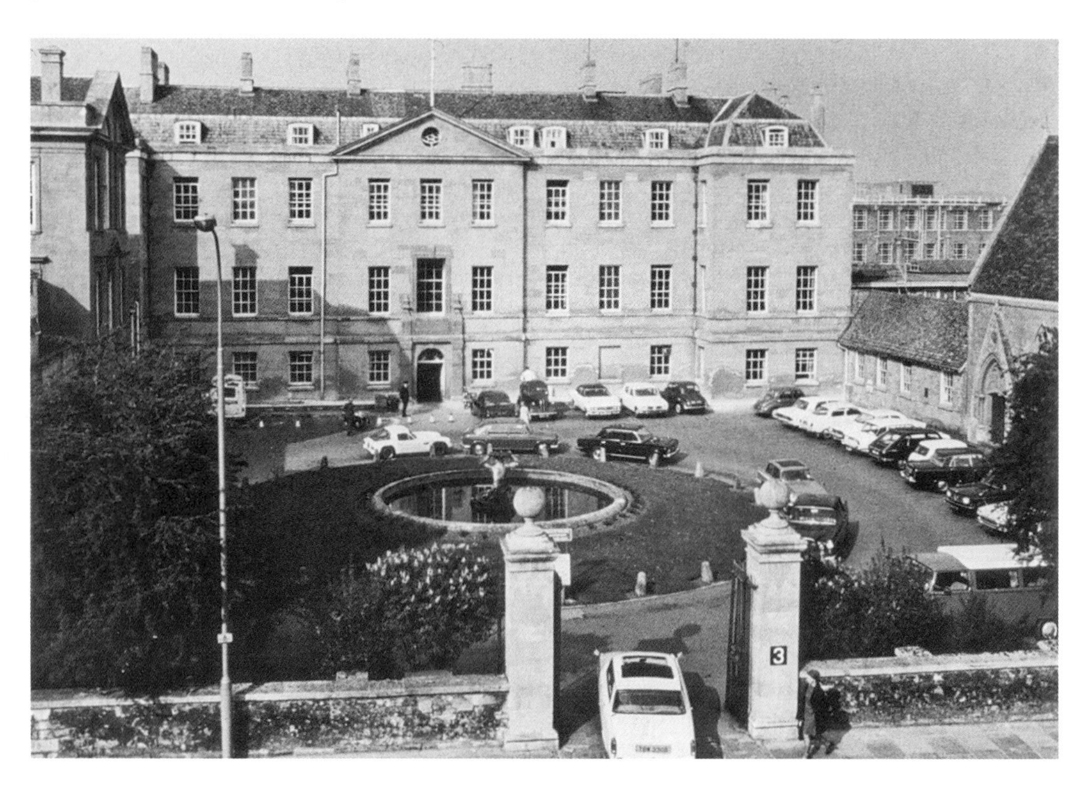

A post-war view: the railings have gone, a contribution to the war effort. By now the motor car has begun to make its impact on the scene.

three

Rules and Records

mixed Caſes of both) whoſe Turn it was to attend, when they were admitted.

67. THAT each Phyſician and Surgeon viſit his reſpective In-Patients, at other Times, as often as he ſhall judge neceſſary, or ſhall have Notice of any ſudden Emergency from the Apotheca---

68. THAT each Phyſician, a
ſineſs or Indiſpoſition ſhall c
engage ſome other Phyſician, o
mary, to attend for him.

69. THAT no Amputation,
ration, be performed in the Infir
Conſultation of all the Phyſicia
ing to it, except on ſome ſudd
ficians and other Surgeons bein

70. THAT the Number of p
not at any Time exceed Six; and that the Number of Surgeons do not exceed Four.

MATRON.

71. THAT the Matron's Salary be Fifteen Pounds a Year; and a Gratuity, not exceeding ten Pounds, be given her if ſhe behaves well.

72. THAT ſhe take Care of all the Houſehold Goods, and Furniture, and be ready to give an Account thereof when required.

73. THAT ſhe keep a daily Account of the Proviſions, and other Neceſſaries, that are brought into the Houſe, and lay it before the Weekly Meeting every *Thurſday*.

74. THAT ſhe take Care, that the Chambers, Beds,

(11)

44. THAT Ladies ſubſcribing as Governors, may vote upon all Occaſions by Proxy under their Hand and Seal. *Ladies may vote by Proxy.*

ADMISSION *and* DISCHARGE *of* PATIENTS.

45. THAT Patients be admitted and diſcharged every *Thurſday* by the Weekly Meeting, between the Hours of Eleven and One. *Time of Admiſſion.*

46. THAT in Caſe a ſufficient Number of Governors cannot be got together, on the Days appointed for the Admiſſion of Patients, it may be lawful for the Phyſician and Surgeon of the Week, with the Conſent of as many Governors as ſhall happen to be preſent, to diſcharge ſuch Patients as deſire to be diſcharged; and alſo to receive into the ſaid Infirmary, ſuch Patients, as ſhall then offer themſelves, and as they ſhall approve of, who are to remain there until the next regular Weekly Meeting determine upon their Admiſſion or Rejection.

47. THAT all Patients who come recommended to the Infirmary, be there before Eleven of the Clock in the Morning on *Thurſdays*, or they cannot be admitted till the Week following.

48. THAT no Patients be admitted, who are able to ſubſiſt themſelves, and pay for Medicines. *Rules of Admiſſion.*

49. THAT no Perſon be admitted a Patient, but by Recommendation of a Subſcriber, or Benefactor, unleſs in Caſes which admit of no Delay; in which Caſes the Apothecary and Matron may receive Patients, giving immediate Notice to the Phyſician or Surgeon of the Week.

50 THAT every Subſcriber, for each Guinea per Ann. ſubſcribed by him, ſhall have a Right to recommend one In-Patient, and one Out-Patient within every

B 2 Year,

(15)

mixed Caſes of both) whoſe Turn it was to attend, when they were admitted.

67. THAT each Phyſician and Surgeon viſit his reſpective In-Patients, at other Times, as often as he ſhall judge neceſſary, or ſhall have Notice of any ſudden Emergency from the Apothecary.

68. THAT each Phyſician, and Surgeon, whoſe Buſineſs or Indiſpoſition ſhall oblige him to be abſent, engage ſome other Phyſician, or Surgeon, of the Infirmary, to attend for him.

69. THAT no Amputation, or other principal Operation, be performed in the Infirmary, without a previous Conſultation of all the Phyſicians and Surgeons belonging to it, except on ſome ſudden Accident, the Phyſicians and other Surgeons being then out of Town.

70. THAT the Number of preſcribing Phyſicians do not at any Time exceed Six; and that the Number of Surgeons do not exceed Four.

MATRON.

71. THAT the Matron's Salary be Fifteen Pounds a Year; and a Gratuity, not exceeding ten Pounds, be given her if ſhe behaves well.

72. THAT ſhe take Care of all the Houſehold Goods, and Furniture, and be ready to give an Account thereof when required.

73. THAT ſhe keep a daily Account of the Proviſions, and other Neceſſaries, that are brought into the Houſe, and lay it before the Weekly Meeting every *Thurſday*.

74. THAT ſhe take Care, that the Chambers, Beds, Clothes, Linen, and all other Things within the Infirmary be kept clean.

75. THAT

Above left: The Radcliffe Infirmary was founded as a charity by those who could afford to pay for a doctor themselves, for the benefit of those who could not. A set of 'Rules and Orders for the Government of the Radcliffe Infirmary' established the criteria for admission (no pregnant women or children under seven except for major surgery) and the procedure whereby subscribers who paid a minimum of 3 guineas a year had a right to recommend patients.

Above right: Stringent requirements were placed on both staff and patients as to their conduct. Patients caught 'smoaking' or swearing could be turned out. Nurses, who were more akin to servants, were required to clean the wards by 7 a.m. in summer and 8 a.m. in winter. And matron, whose duties were those of a housekeeper more than a leader of a profession, kept the books and ordered the food.

This page also shows the requirement of a joint consultation between surgeons and physicians before major surgery was performed, a ruling which irked many of the more confident surgeons 100 years later and was abandoned before the First World War.

1797 Jan 31 John Bryant of Kirtlington (37)

Ae. 17 Oc. Sept 6

has been in ye House since Jan. 19 – is affected with nervous Symptoms – Giddiness, frights, tremblings, sometimes amounting to a fit, but his appetite good, his Sleep natural, his Body regular – &c – Applic. Emplast. Canth. larg. Capiti raso – Capiat Pil. [illegible] also [illegible] ter die – Mist. [illegible] Valer. [illegible]

Feb 2 The Blister has risen well, & he says, has relieved his Head – Has had no fit but has not slept so well as usual – Other Symptoms nearly ye same as above – Medicines again &c.

Feb 5 Has been particularly Dull heavy & cold – He neither any positive fit. P. 75 – Extremities cold – Had a stool [illegible] day (irregularly) – Ry Conf. Arom. [illegible] Aq. Menth. [illegible] [illegible] Amm. [illegible] gtt xxx [illegible] 4tis Horis

12 Has been better for some Days – his Head more clear & Spirits improved – but to-day seems again more Dull & heavy – Body regular – Appetite & Sleep natural – – Ry Conf. Arom. [illegible] Aq. Menth. [illegible] Tinct. Valer. [illegible] sextis Horis

13 Thinks himself much better – is more clear in his Head, more awake & cheerful – P. 84 sufficiently strong – regular in his Body, &c & his Medicines again &c

14 Not quite so well to-day – more confused, dull & heavy – speaks of fluttering &c in his Stomach – Body regular – Skin cold & [illegible] – Pulse [illegible] – Repet. Med. [illegible] Quantitate T. Valerian ad [illegible]

16 Has been more lively & cheerful since our last Visit & appears to be in general good Health with respect to all ye natural Functions – but is still slow & heavy in his Head – Applicetur [illegible] Emplast. Cantharid. [illegible] – & [illegible] in Med.

18 The Blister has done its Duty – His Head seems a little upon my [illegible] – Body regular – Capiat Pulv. Rad. Valer. [illegible] ter die in Mist. [illegible]

Case histories – records of each case were handwritten in a large volume. This entry records the treatment of John Bryant, of Kirtlington, in 1797, who was admitted with, 'severe symptoms of giddiness, frights, tremblings, sometimes amounting to fits'. He was treated by 'blistering' – raising the skin by application of heated glass or chemicals – which the record says relieved his head. After about two weeks he told the doctors he felt better and desired to go home.

The Register of Operations. In 1838 the Quarterly Court of the Infirmary resolved that a book should be provided, 'in which an entry is to be made of each operation immediately after it has been performed, with such observations as the case may suggest'.

This entry records the case of a twelve-year-old boy, George Harris, who was driving horses harrowing a field at Headington in March 1850 when a horse became restive, knocked him down and a harrow tine struck him on the head. 'The blow did not render him insensible and he walked all the way to the Infirmary almost immediately.' Surgeon Mr Hussey performed the operation of 'trepanning' on his badly damaged skull and three months later he was discharged cured.

Industrial injuries were also common. In this case from June 1847, Mr Hitchings amputated the right forearm of John Horwood of St Giles, aged thirteen, whose hand was drawn into a printing machine, pulling the skin off like a glove turned inside out. In an early example of anaesthetics it records that vapour of ether was inhaled with complete success.

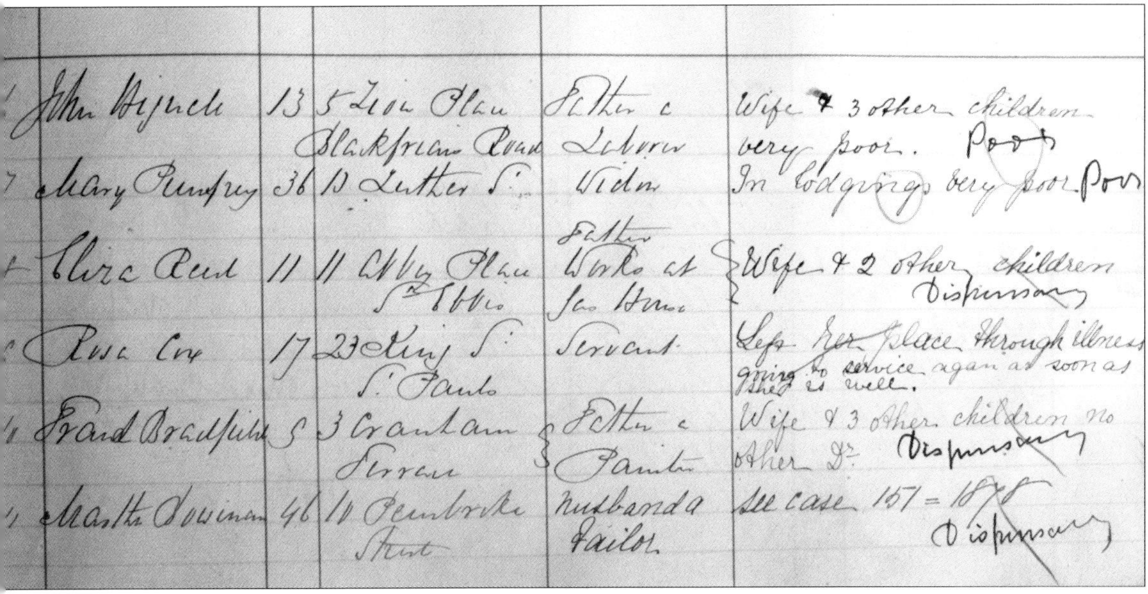

John Hignell	13	5 Zion Place Blackfriars Road	Father a Laborer	Wife & 3 other children very poor. Poor
Mary Rumfrey	36	13 Luther St	Widow	In lodgings very poor. Poor
Eliza Reed	11	11 Abbey Place St Ebbes	Father Works at Gas Works	Wife & 2 other children Dispensary
Rose Cox	17	23 King St St Pauls	Servant	Left her place through illness going to service again as soon as she is well.
Frank Bradfield	5	3 Cranham Terrace	Father a Painter	Wife & 3 other children no other Dr. Dispensary
Martha Dossiman	46	10 Pembroke Street	Husband a Tailor	See case 157 = 1878 Dispensary

Above: The provident dispensary. In 1877 a provident dispensary was founded in Oxford. As the Infirmary was for the relief of the poor, the governors felt they could now 'with propriety' refuse treatment to people who ought to have made themselves members of the dispensary.

Enquiries were made about people seeking admission as to their fitness as objects of charitable relief. The first two recorded here were deemed to be genuinely poor – and therefore suitable. The last three were referred to the dispensary. The book is in Oxfordshire Health Archives.

Right: The minute books. Minutes of the meetings of the committee of governors were recorded in bound books in exemplary copperplate handwriting from 1770 until the hospital joined the NHS in 1948. They are a model of terse but eloquent style. This extract, from 1877, records the special court of governors, presided over by Prince Leopold, at which the gift of the new children's ward from Martha Combe was acknowledged.

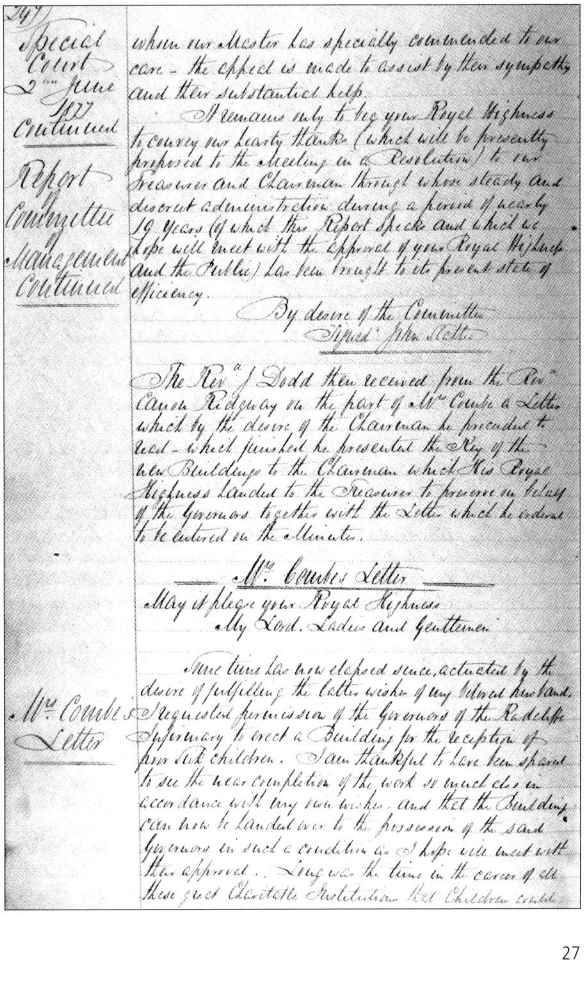

247

Special Court 2nd June 1877 Continued

whom our Master has specially commended to our care – the appeal is made to assist by their sympathy and their substantial help.

It remains only to beg your Royal Highness to convey our hearty thanks (which will be presently proposed to the Meeting in a Resolution) to our Treasurer and Chairman through whose steady and discreet administration during a period of nearly 19 years (of which this Report speaks and which we hope will meet with the approval of your Royal Highness and the Public) has been brought to its present state of efficiency.

Report Committee of Management Continued

By desire of the Committee
Signed John Slatter

The Revd J Dodd then received from the Revd Canon Ridgway on the part of Mrs Combe a Letter which by the desire of the Chairman he proceeded to read – which finished he presented the Key of the new Buildings to the Chairman which His Royal Highness handed to the Treasurer to preserve on behalf of the Governors together with the Letter which he ordered to be entered on the Minutes.

Mrs Combe's Letter

May it please your Royal Highness
My Lord, Ladies and Gentlemen

Mrs Combe's Letter

Some time has now elapsed since, actuated by the desire of fulfilling the latter wishes of my beloved husband, I requested permission of the Governors of the Radcliffe Infirmary to erect a Building for the reception of poor sick children. I am thankful to have been spared to see the near completion of the work so much else in accordance with my own wishes – and that the Building can now be handed over to the possession of the said Governors in such a condition as I hope will meet with their approval. Long was the time in the career of all these great Charitable Institutions that Children could

6 Carlton Gardens
Ap. 23. 1849.

Sir

I have recd the report of the Radcliffe Infirmary this morning and I see my name entered as a Subscriber of Forty Guineas. But on the 3d of July last my Bankers Sir S. Scott and Co paid my cheque for fifty guineas in favour of the Infirmary. Will you have the goodness to examine this matter

Left: Where's my cash? William Gladstone, MP and later Prime Minister, was a regular supporter of the hospital and sent the governors 50 guineas in 1848. But when the annual report came out in 1849 it showed him as a subscriber of only 40 guineas. ('But on the 3rd of July last my Bankers Sir S Scott and Co paid my cheque for fifty guineas in favour of the Infirmary', he wrote. 'Will you have the goodness to examine this matter.')

Below: 'No curtains', says Florence. In 1863 the hospital was considering putting curtains round the beds and wrote to Florence Nightingale for advice on how to hang them. Her reply was robust and uncompromising. 'As the conviction of my hospital life has been that no curtains should be allowed to come near any hospital bedstead to obstruct its fresh air, I cannot advise on how to hang curtains', she writes. If the patient needed privacy, staff should use low movable screens.

As the conviction of my Hospital life has been that no curtains should be allowed to come near any Hospital bedstead, to obstruct its fresh air, I cannot advise on how to hang curtains. If the Patient requires privacy, low moveable screens should be used just high enough to prevent him seeing into other beds or other beds seeing into him, i.e. not higher than the Patient's head when sitting up in

four

Victorian and Edwardian

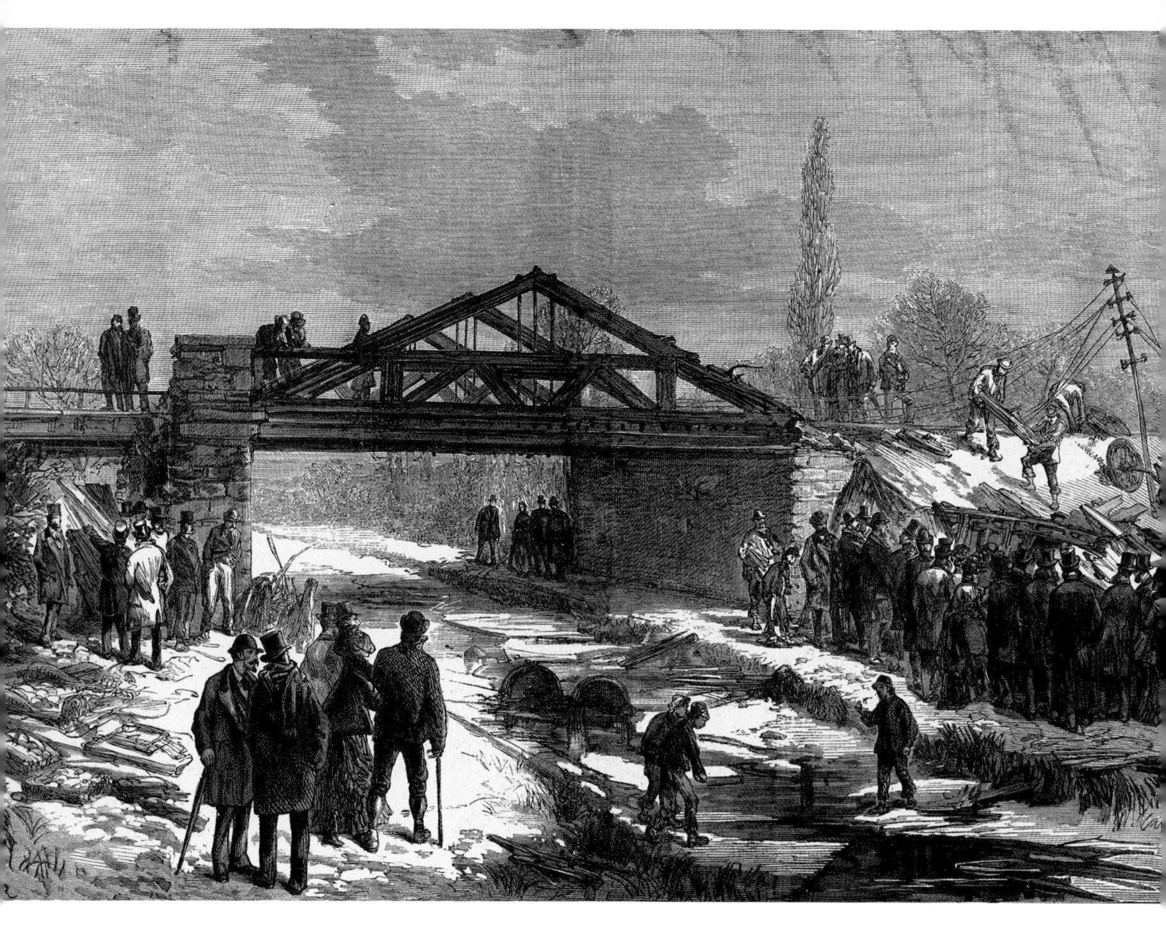

The Shipton-on-Cherwell train crash. On Christmas Eve 1874 the express train from Paddington to Birkenhead left Oxford at 12.15 p.m. with an extra engine and carriages added. As the train approached Hampton Gay, several carriages left the rails and were shattered as they plunged down the embankment near the Oxford canal.

Twenty-six people died at the scene and others later, bringing the total to thirty-four, the worst rail disaster in history at the time. A special train was sent to bring the injured back to Oxford and fifty of them were taken through the streets on stretchers to the Radcliffe Infirmary. Others, according to their means and injuries, went to colleges and hotels.

The house surgeon, William Morgan, led a team of doctors who worked long into the night treating the injured, many of whom were, 'profoundly comatose and benumbed with cold, their clothes stiff and frozen and their limbs fixed and rigid. Nearly all were suffering from shock and a large number had sustained fractures ... scarcely one person had escaped without severe laceration of some part of the body.'

The severity of the incident prompted Queen Victoria to order a telegram to be sent to ask how the injured were progressing and donations by the public and by the Great Western Railway (who gave £250), 'profoundly influenced the financial situation of the institution'. (*Illustrated London News*)

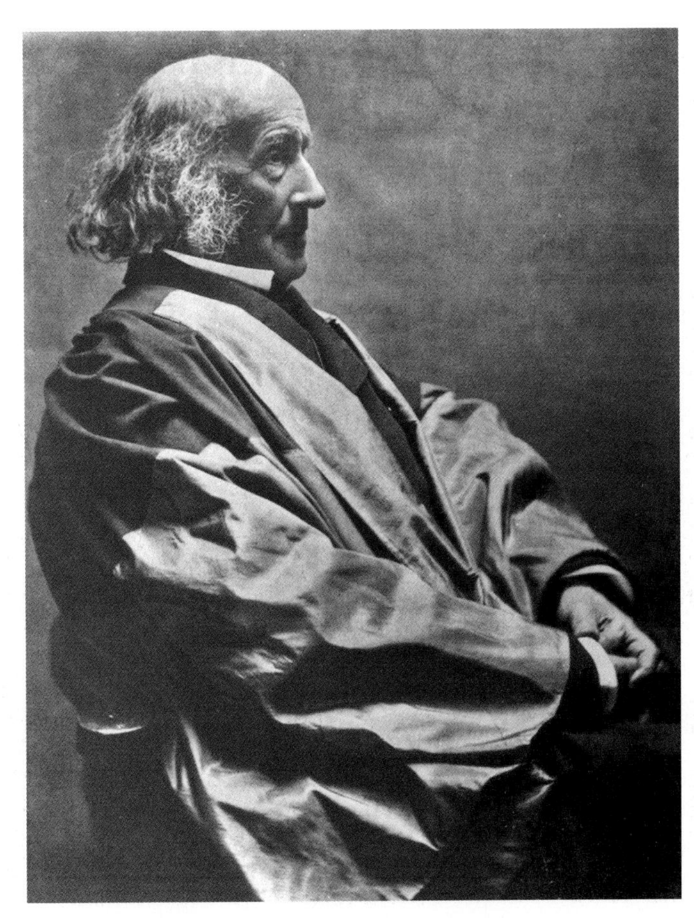

Sir Henry Acland 1815-1900 Physician to the Infirmary in 1847-79 and Regius Professor of Medicine, University of Oxford 1857-95, he was a dominant force in the affairs of both in the late nineteenth century. He was a pioneer (so far as Oxford was concerned) in the use of diagnostic instruments like the stethoscope and microscope and an 'effective man of business' with vision. In the cholera epidemic in Oxford in 1854 he did much to control an outbreak that threatened more lives than the 116 who died.

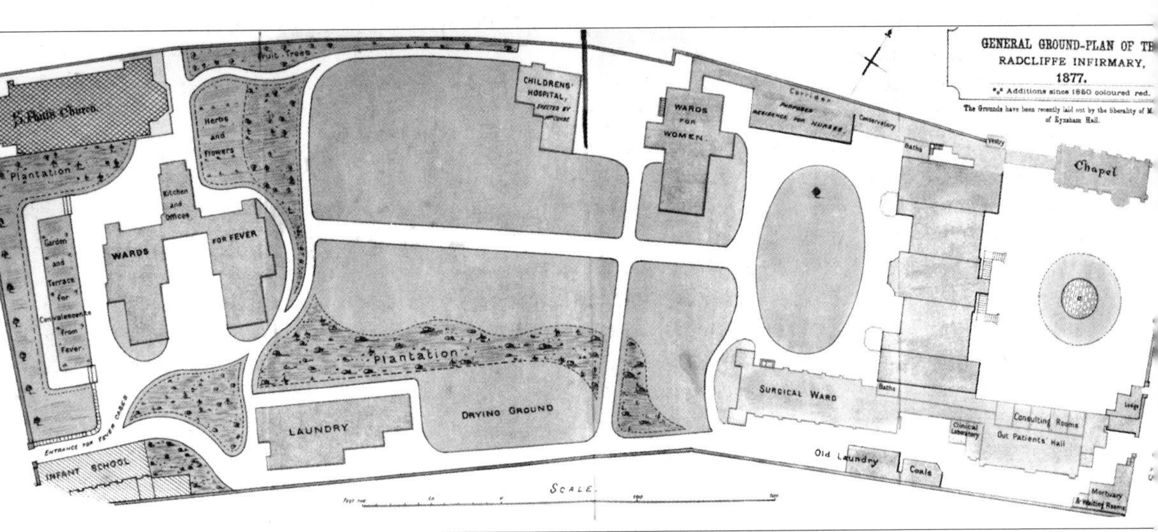

The layout of the site in 1877 showing the original outpatients hall (bottom right), the children's hospital (top centre), the fever hospital – later the Oxford Eye Hospital – (left, near St Paul's Church) and the chapel (top right).

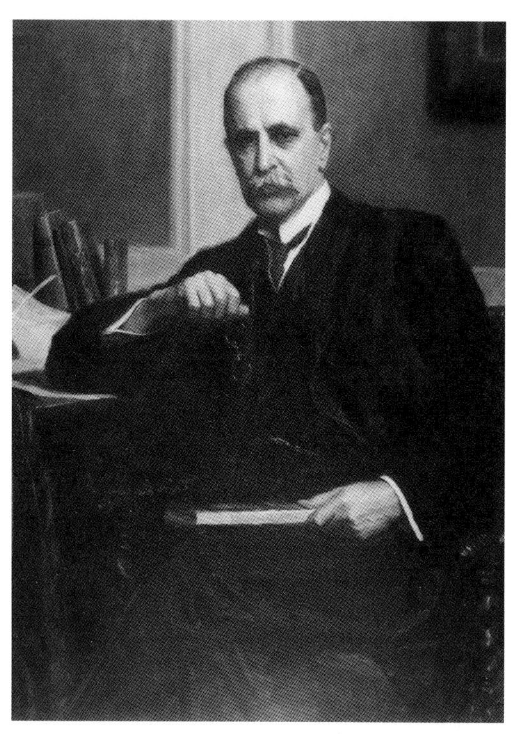

Left: Sir William Osler 1849-1919
He was perhaps the most famous and most admired of the Regius Professors, who came to Oxford in 1905 after a very distinguished career in medicine and teaching in his native Canada and in the United States. His book *Principles and Practice of Medicine* (1892) won international acclaim.

Many photographs show him looking severely over his heavy moustache, but he was in fact a warm-hearted man with a twinkle in his eye who radiated an infectious enthusiasm and was much loved by his students and professional colleagues. His home in Norham Gardens was known as 'The Open Arms' because of the welcome extended to so many.

Below: Osler at the bedside – a picture taken during his time at Johns Hopkins University in Baltimore. His reputation as a bedside teacher was one of the reasons he was invited to Oxford.

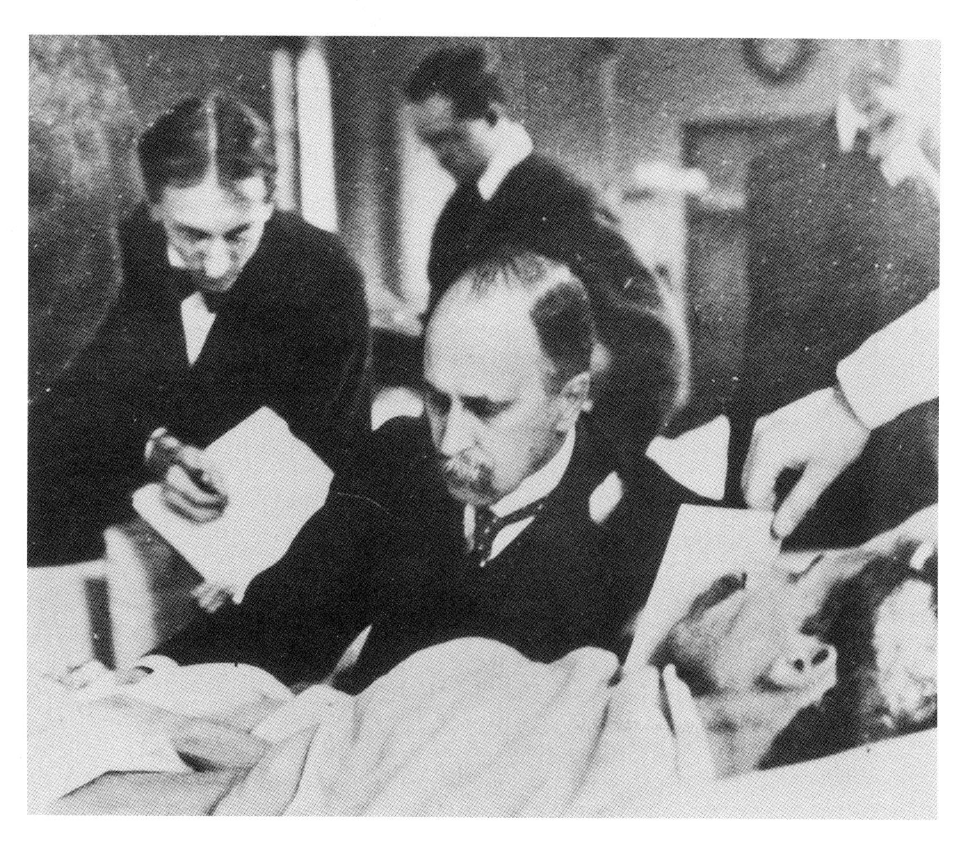

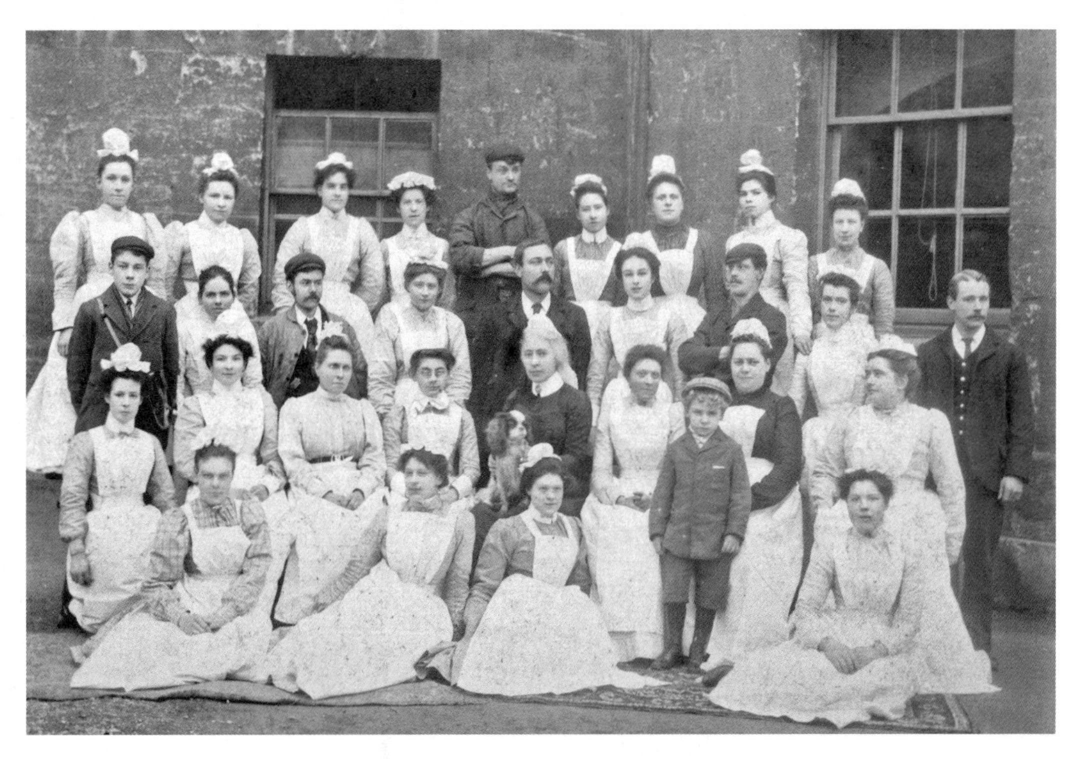

One of the few surviving pictures which shows both nursing and other staff, *c.* 1900. The matron in the centre is thought to be Agnes Watt, described by Robb-Smith as quite definitely the head of the hospital with a fine bosom and close-fitting dress who would sail around the hospital with a regal demeanour. The reputation of her training school was high and she insisted on high standards of behaviour.

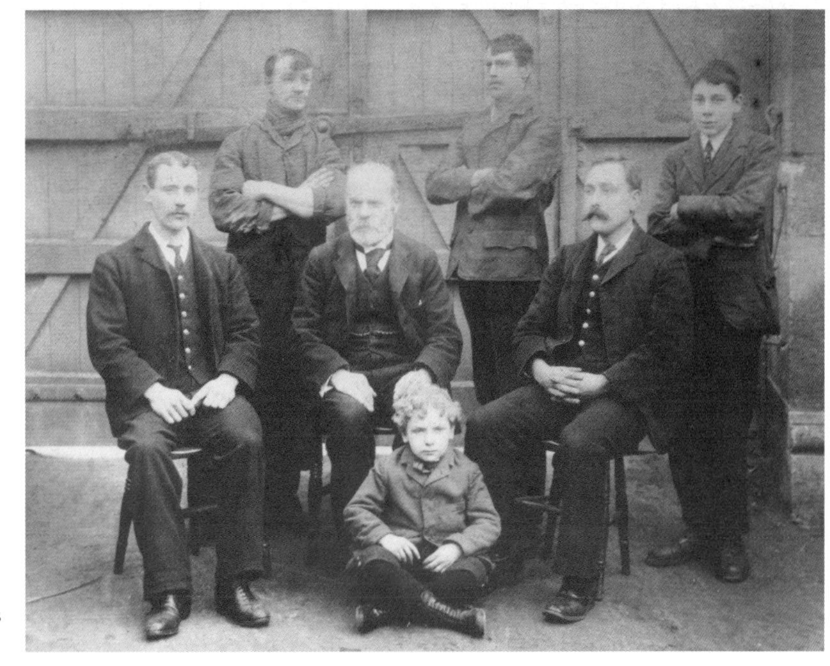

A group of porters, *c.* 1900. The small boy in the front appears to feature in the picture above as well.

The next six pictures are from an album of photographs by Margaret 'Nellie' Anderson who was assistant matron for over twenty-five years before she resigned in 1919 and went to live in Canada. The pictures are from around 1900–10.

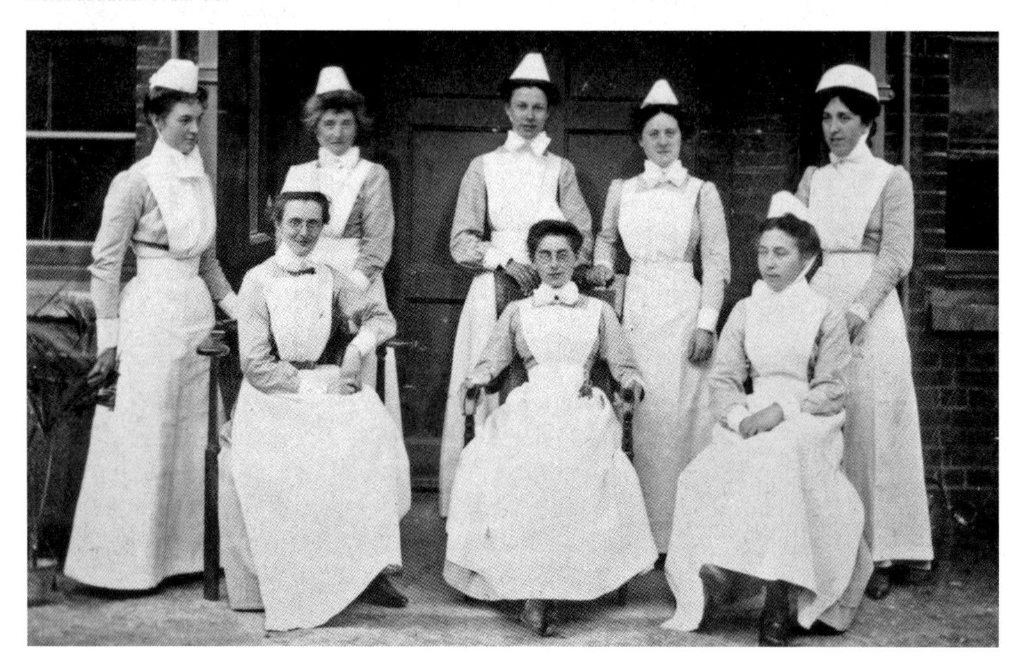

Nellie Anderson (centre) with nursing colleagues.

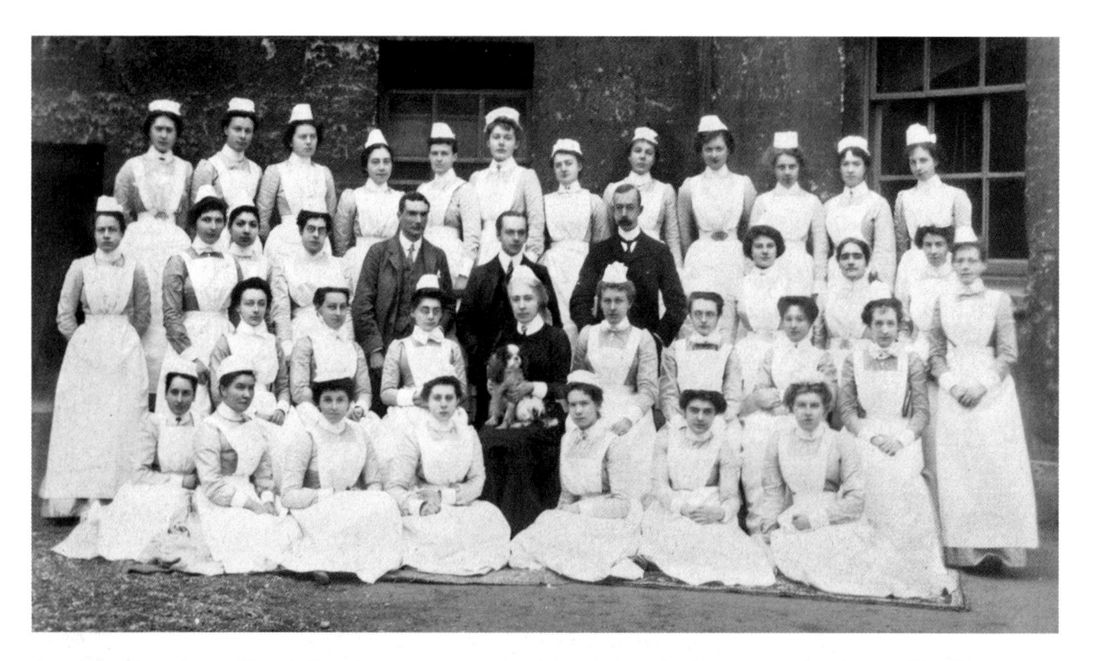

A group of nursing staff including the matron, Agnes Watt (centre, with her dog on her lap) and Nellie sitting on her right. The men in the picture may be the 'house doctors' who were paid by the hospital. The senior physicians held honorary posts and were in private practice outside.

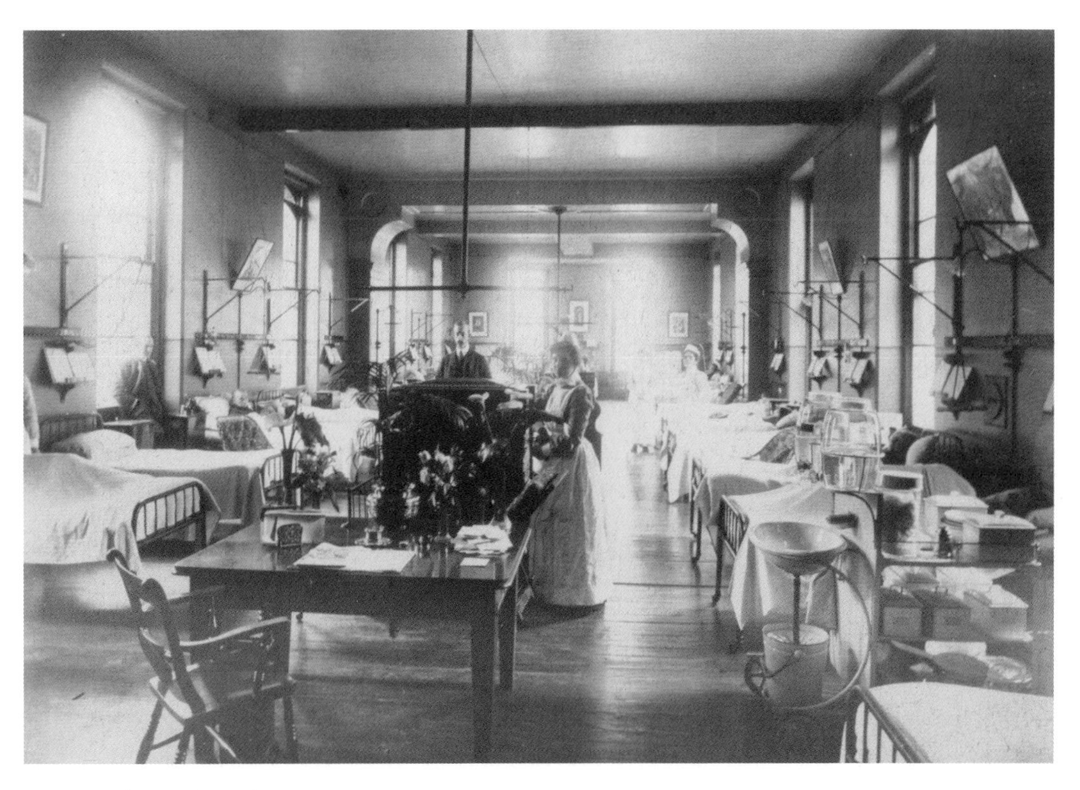

Marlborough ward.

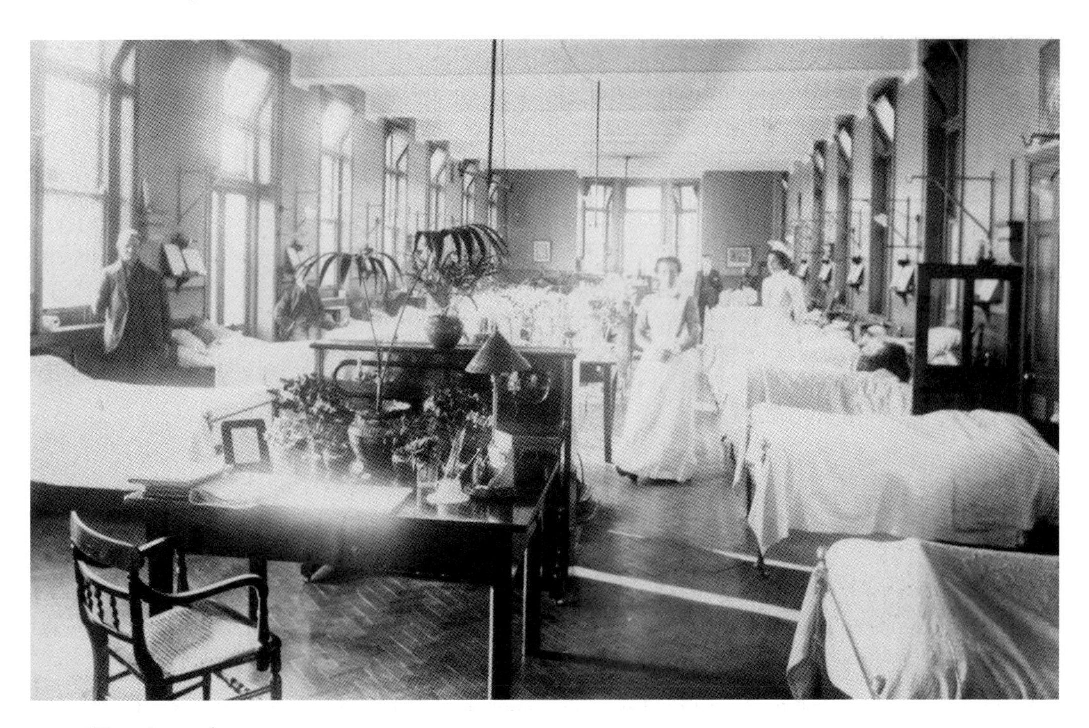

Victoria ward.

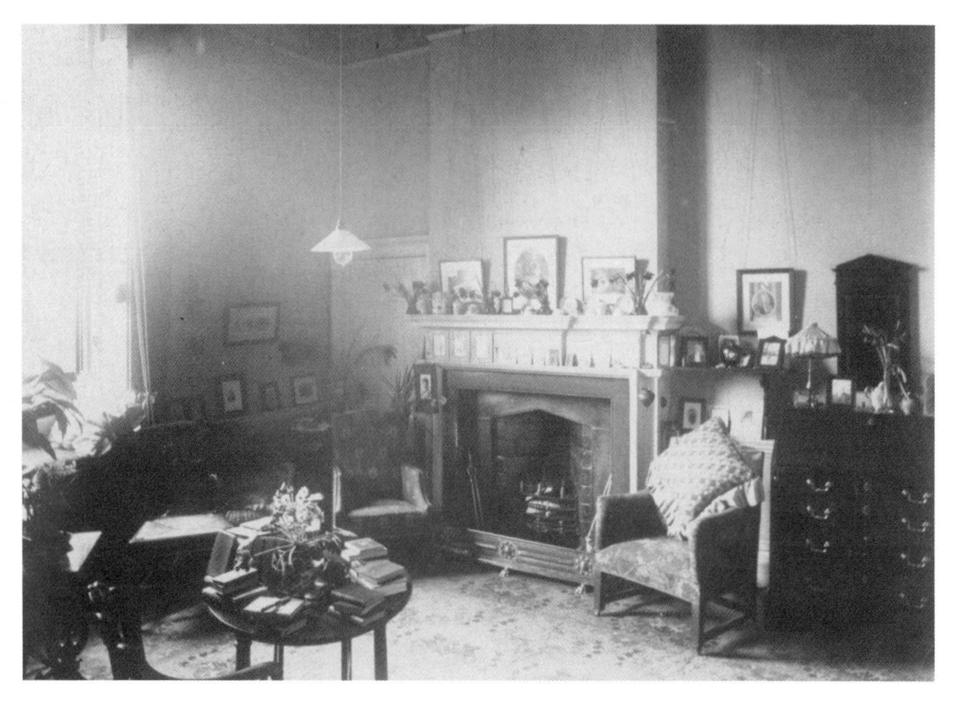

This picture is captioned simply 'my room' in Nellie's album. Both Nellie and the matron had their own rooms and would have spent most of their lives living in the hospital.

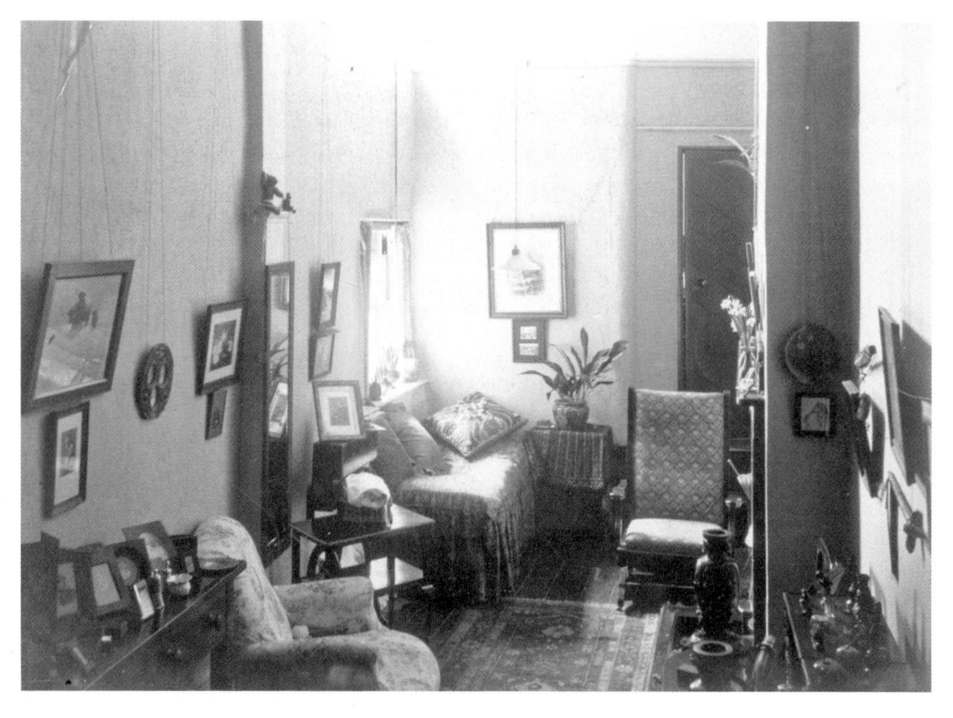

Matron's sitting room. Agnes Watt dispensed dignified hospitality here and surgeons and physicians would take a glass of sherry after ward rounds or operations.

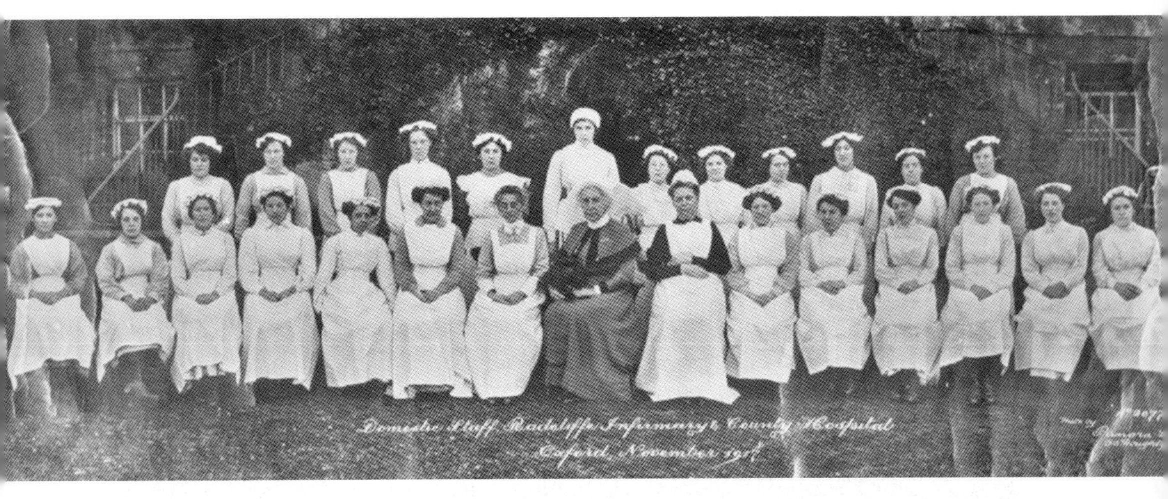

The domestic staff in 1917. From left to right, front row: Gladys Bradley, Harris, Woods, Gertrude Whiting, Nancy, Wildman (Head Laundress), Margaret Anderson (Assistant Matron), Agnes Watt (Matron), Mrs Watkins, -?- , -?- , -?- , Woods, King, Beal. Back row: Woods, -?- , King, Franklin, Savins (Matron's Maid). The remainder are unknown. The three Woods were sisters.

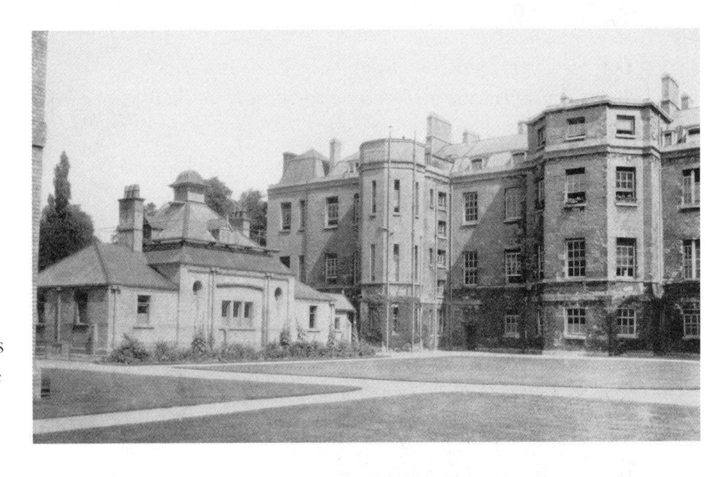

The new operating theatre (left) in 1909. It opened in 1899 on the site of the original fever ward. When the hospital opened 130 years previously, surgery took place on the top floor of the main building.

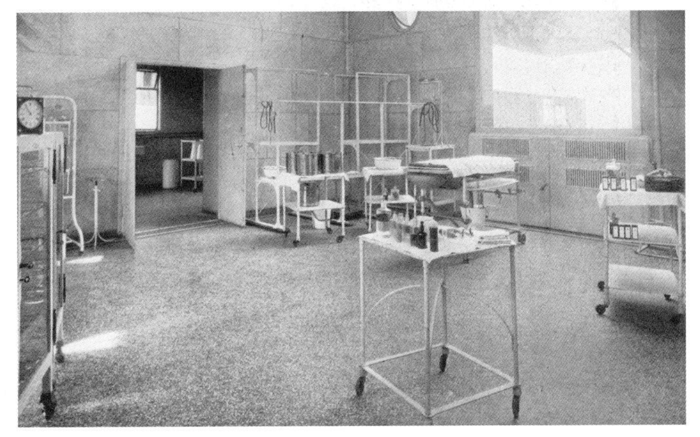

Inside the operating theatre, *c.* 1907.

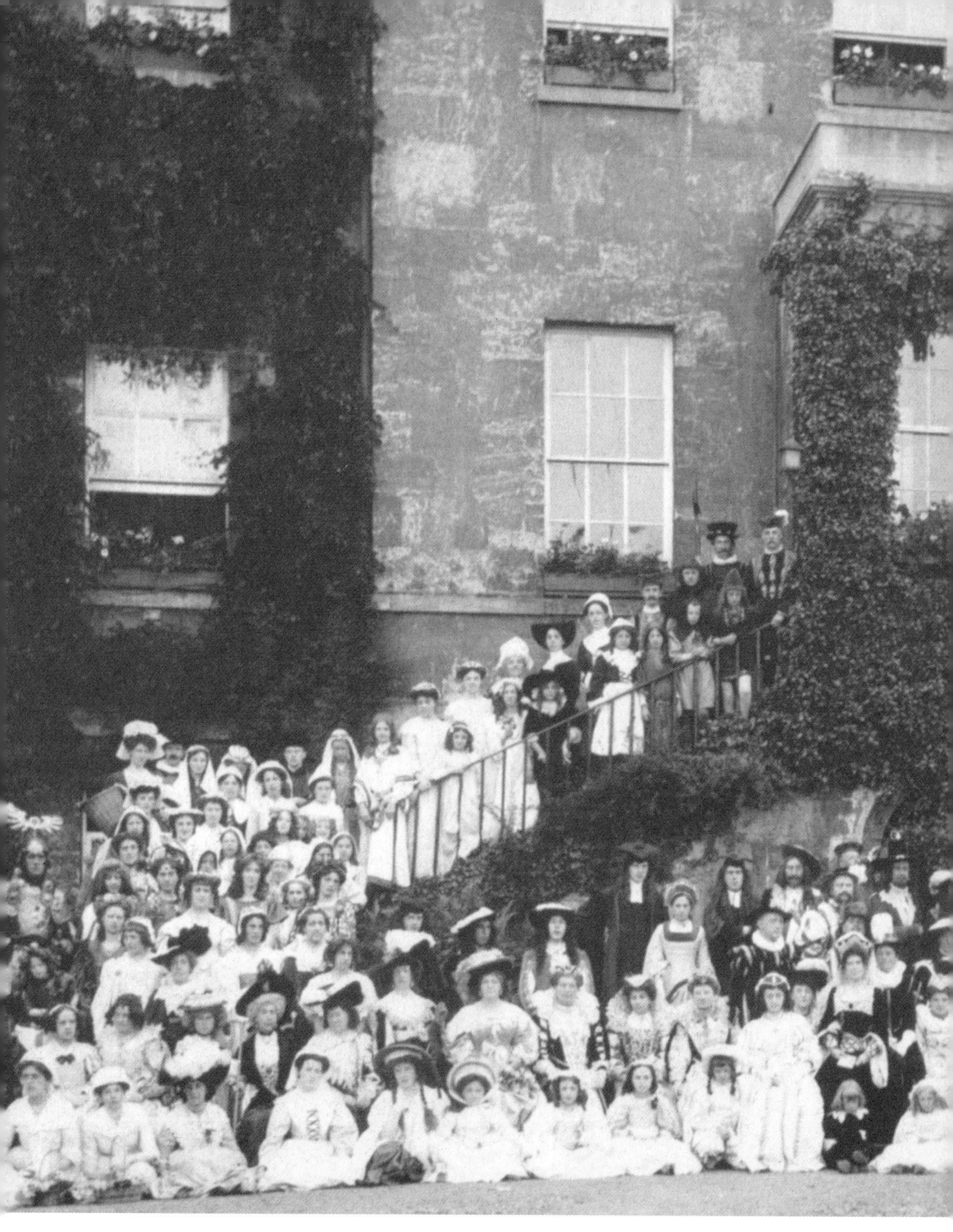

The Oxford Historical Pageant. In midsummer 1907 a committee of supporters staged the Oxford Historical Pageant in aid of the Infirmary and the Eye Hospital. It took place at the end of the Broad Walk near the banks of the Cherwell and featured a 'pomp of picturesque ceremonial' depicting major events in Oxford's history.

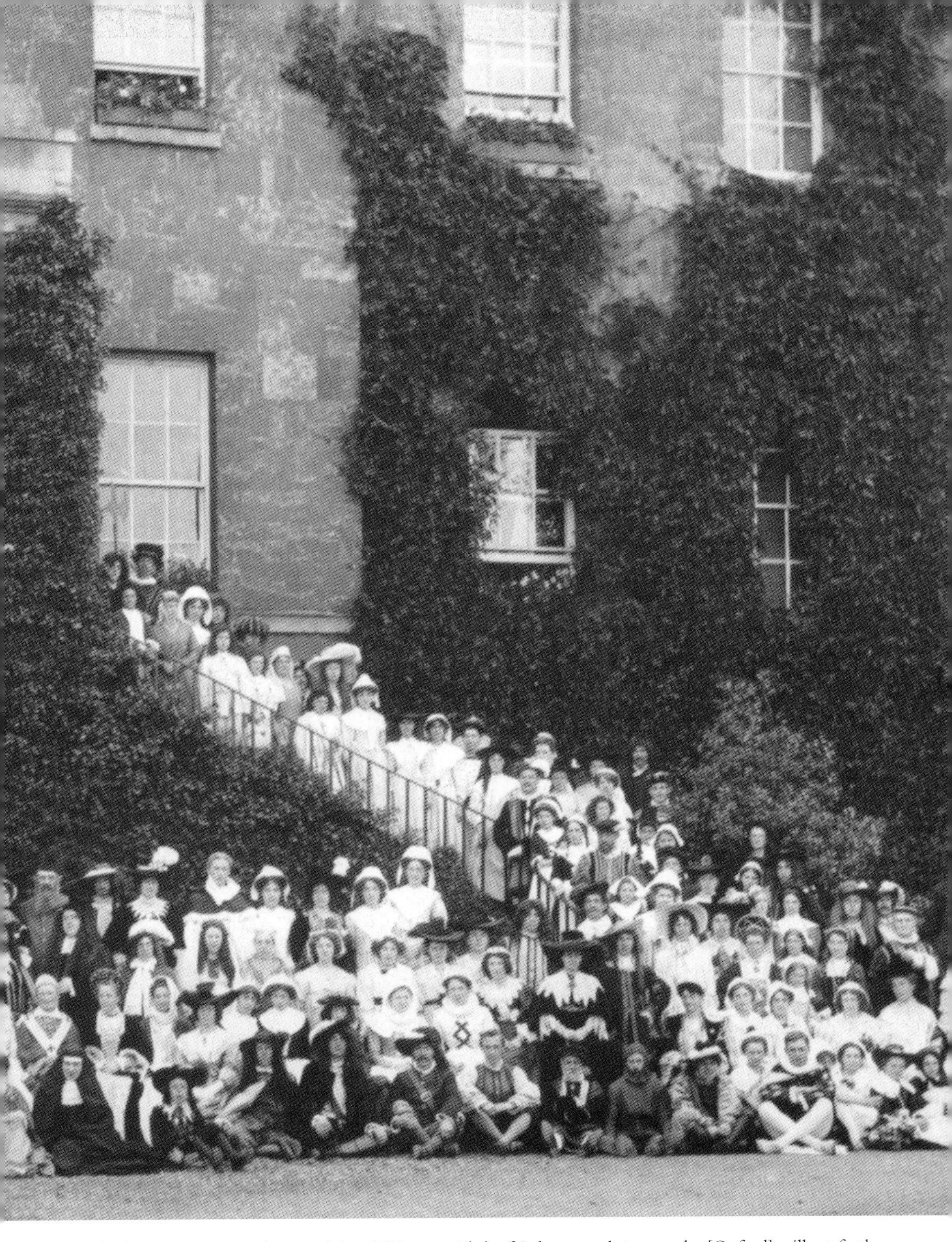

As the programme writer proclaimed, 'Here, amid the fair lawns and streams she [Oxford] will set forth, brilliant and unclouded as when they first met her gaze, the noblest memories of a thousand years.' RI staff joined enthusiastically in the project and were among the cast who posed for this picture on the front stairs.

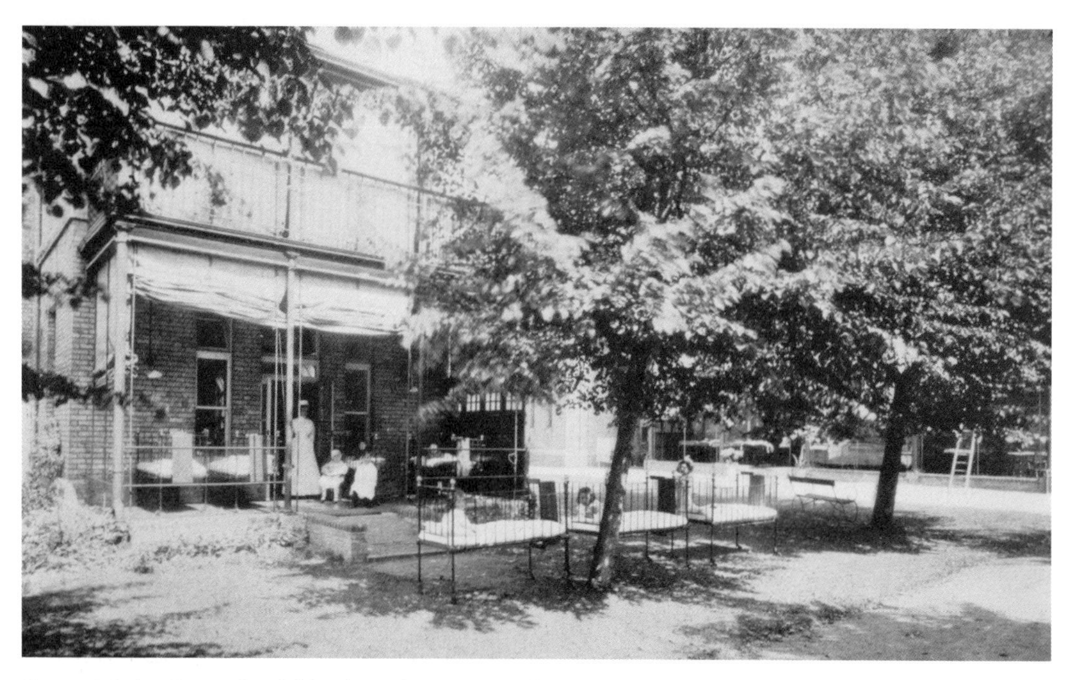

Open-air balconies on the children's ward in 1909. Fresh air was very much part of the treatment for all types of patients.

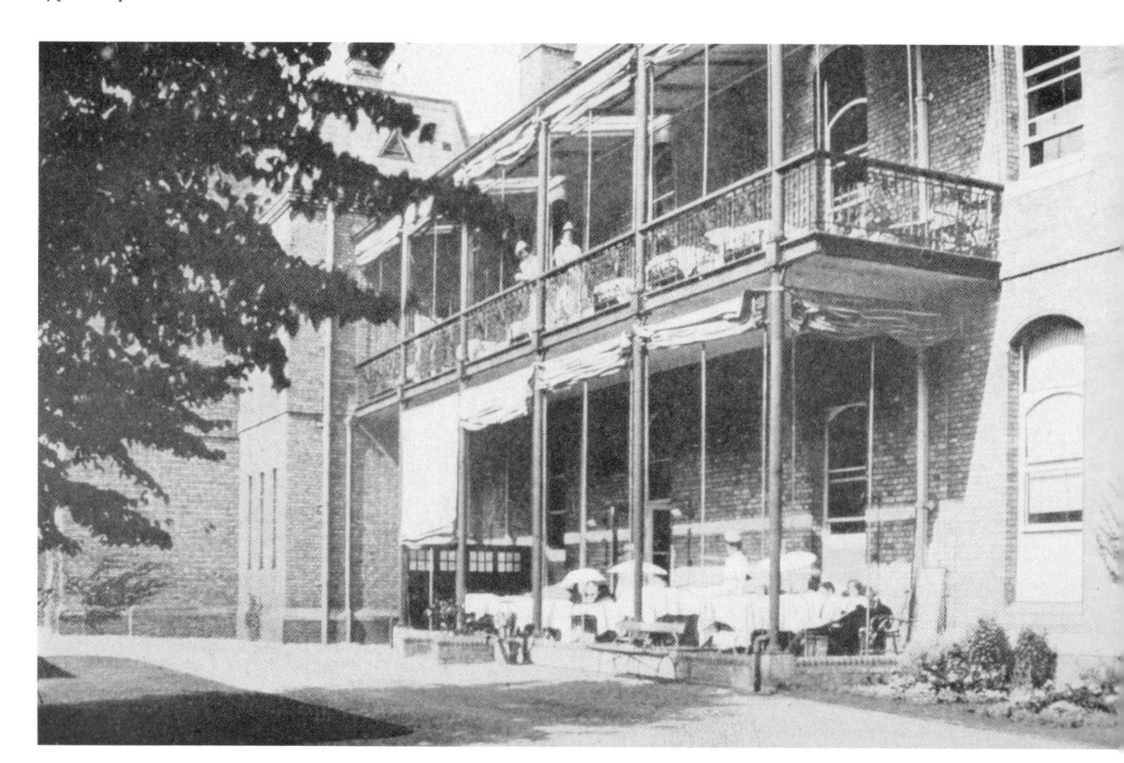

Patients enjoy the sunshine on the balconies of Victoria and Alexandra wards in 1911.

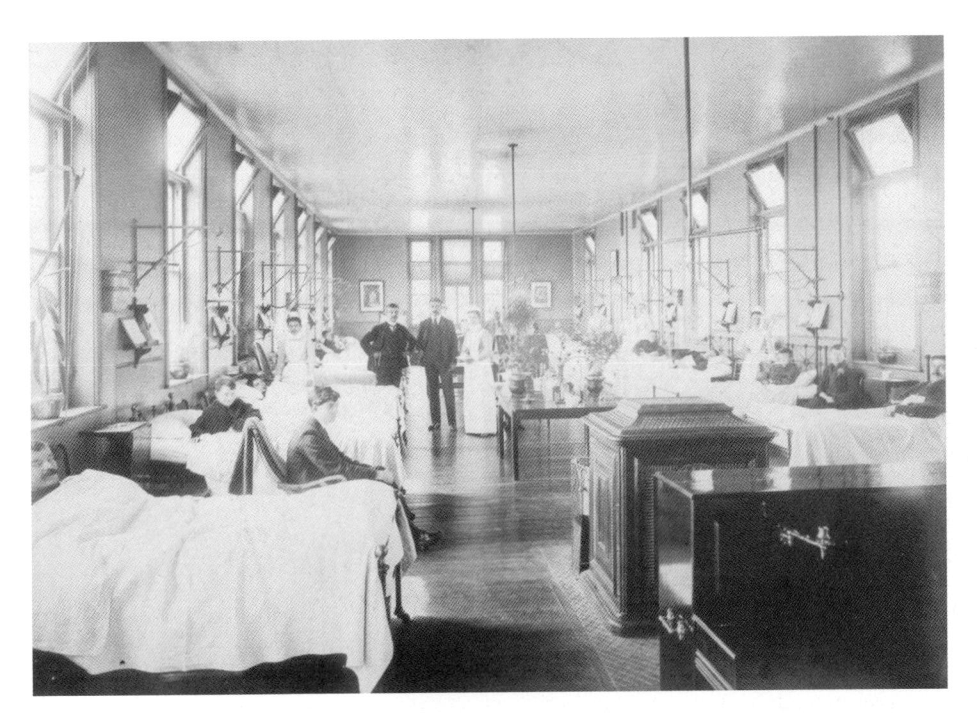

Rowney ward complete with piano and elegant furniture, *c.* 1900.

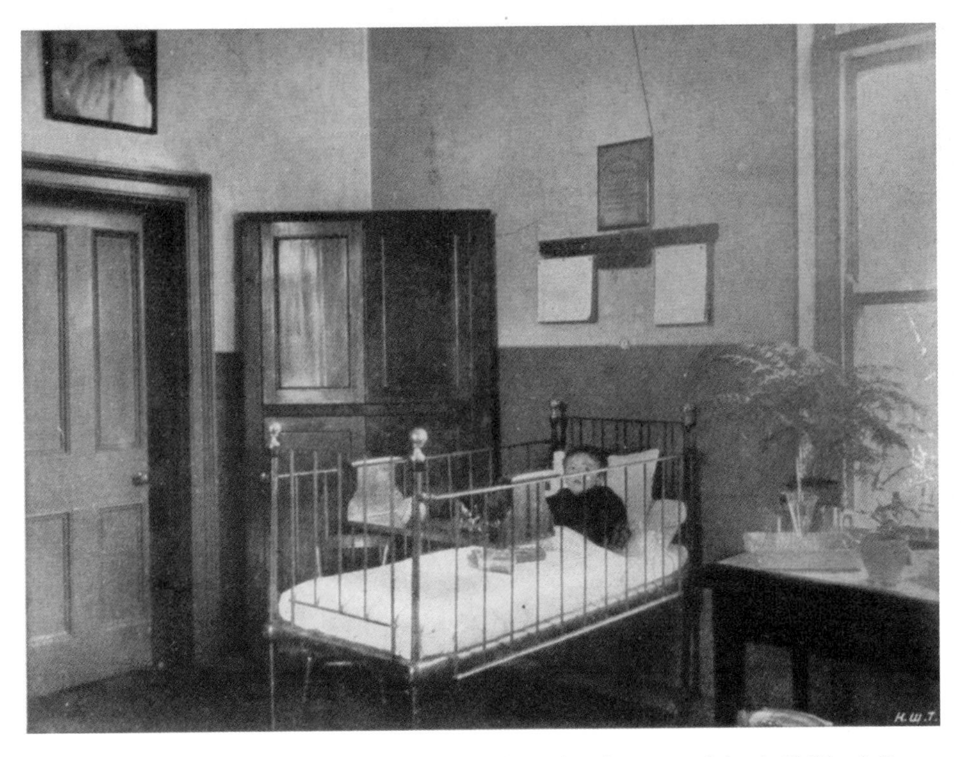

The Infirmary was sustained by charity – this time from the Elementary Schools Children's Cot Association which proudly photographed 'our cot' in the children's ward.

During the First World War Somerville College became part of the Third Southern General Hospital and was well supported by the skills of staff and the scientific resources of the neighbouring Infirmary. A gateway was knocked in the wall between the two to allow the easy flow of staff and equipment. A similar exercise took place during the Second World War when Somerville also accommodated medical students evacuated from London hospitals.

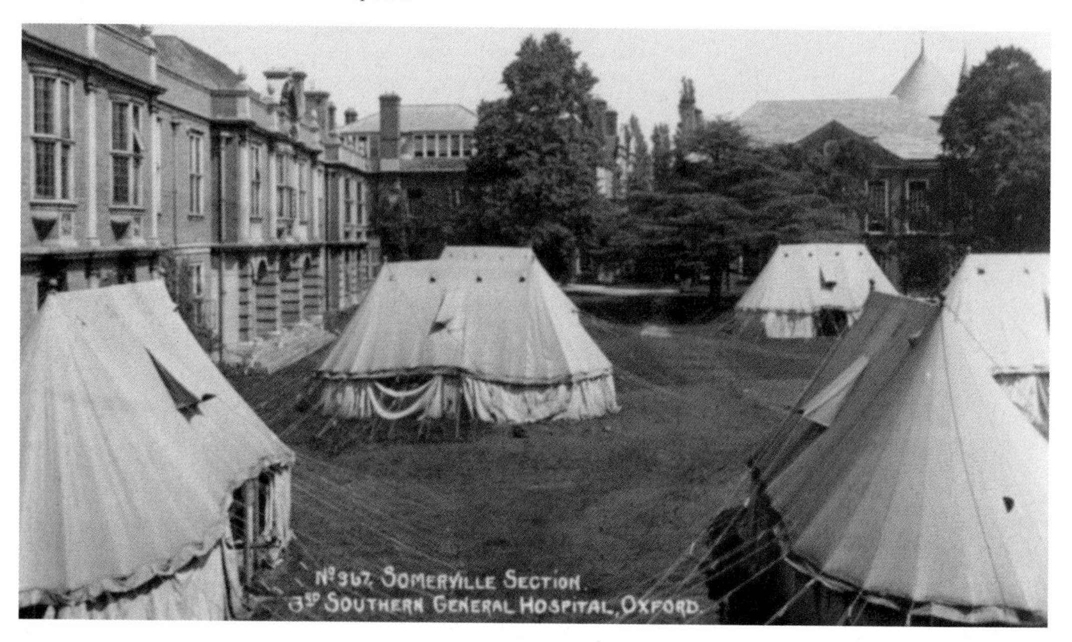

Above: Tents in the quadrangle. (Somerville College)

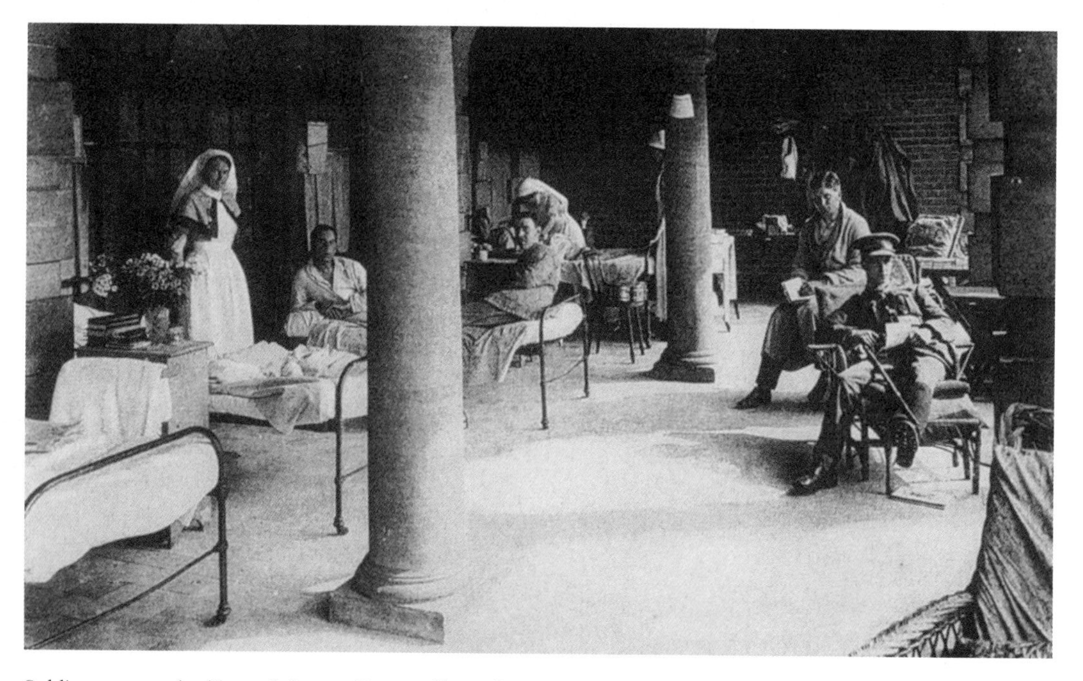

Soldiers rest on the library balcony. (Somerville College)

five

Between the Wars

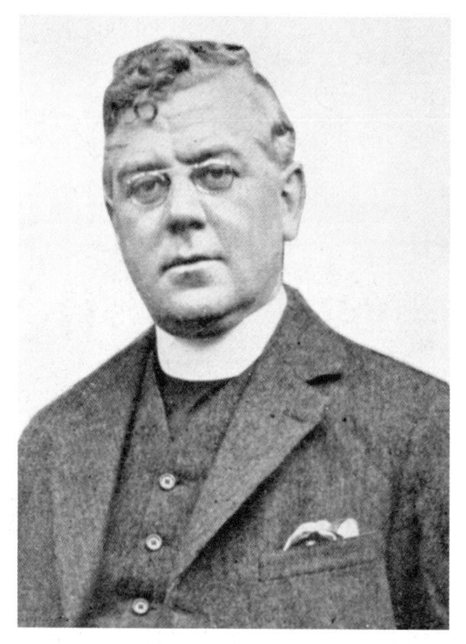

The Revd George Cronshaw 1872-1929
He was treasurer from 1910 to 1928 and responsible for perhaps one of the boldest decisions in the hospital's history when he persuaded the governors to buy the Manor House site in 1919, on which the John Radcliffe Hospital now stands. The manor and 140 acres cost £16,000. It was desperately needed to relieve overcrowding and to provide a sanatorium for tuberculosis patients.

A man of vision and ceaseless energy, Cronshaw was also bursar and tutor in chemistry at the Queen's College and a great *bon viveur*. He travelled everywhere by foot or bike and argued that the soundest way to raise money was to do the job well and ask for money later.

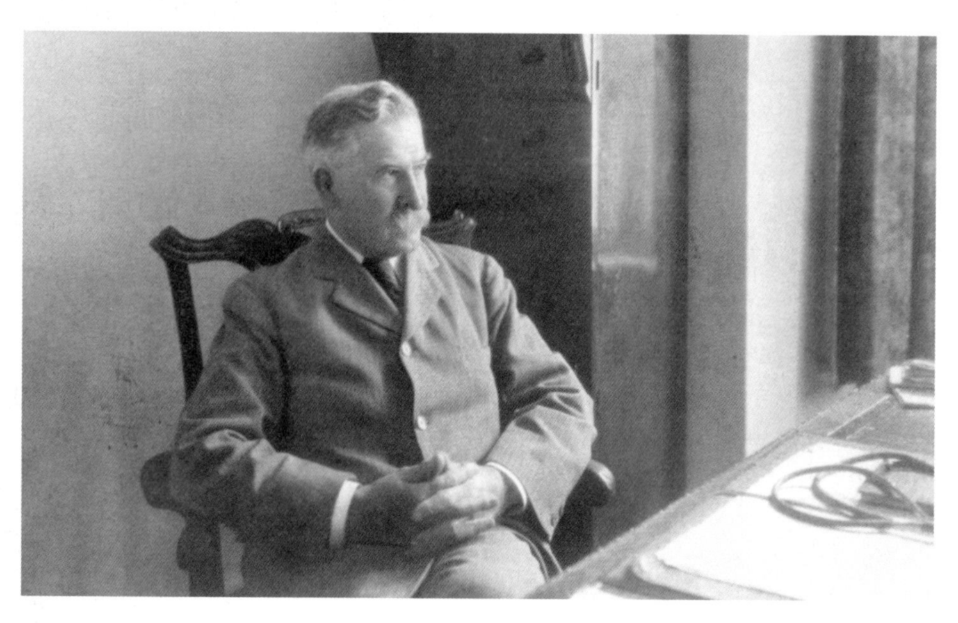

Dr William Collier 1856-1935
He was house physician in 1881 and honorary physician from 1885 to 1921. On his retirement he became a member of the committee of management. In 1920 he suggested a scheme for people to contribute 2*d* a week and he and other staff toured the towns and villages of Oxfordshire to promote the idea. Within three years it was contributing 60 per cent of the hospital's income.

Robb-Smith describes him as a man of strong opinions, argumentative and straightforward with an underlying kindly and sympathetic nature. He was as interested in the policy and management of the hospital as he was in his medical work and as concerned for its reputation and prosperity as he was of his own. A keen and able sportsman, he also rode a motorbike until his family sold the machine to make him stop.

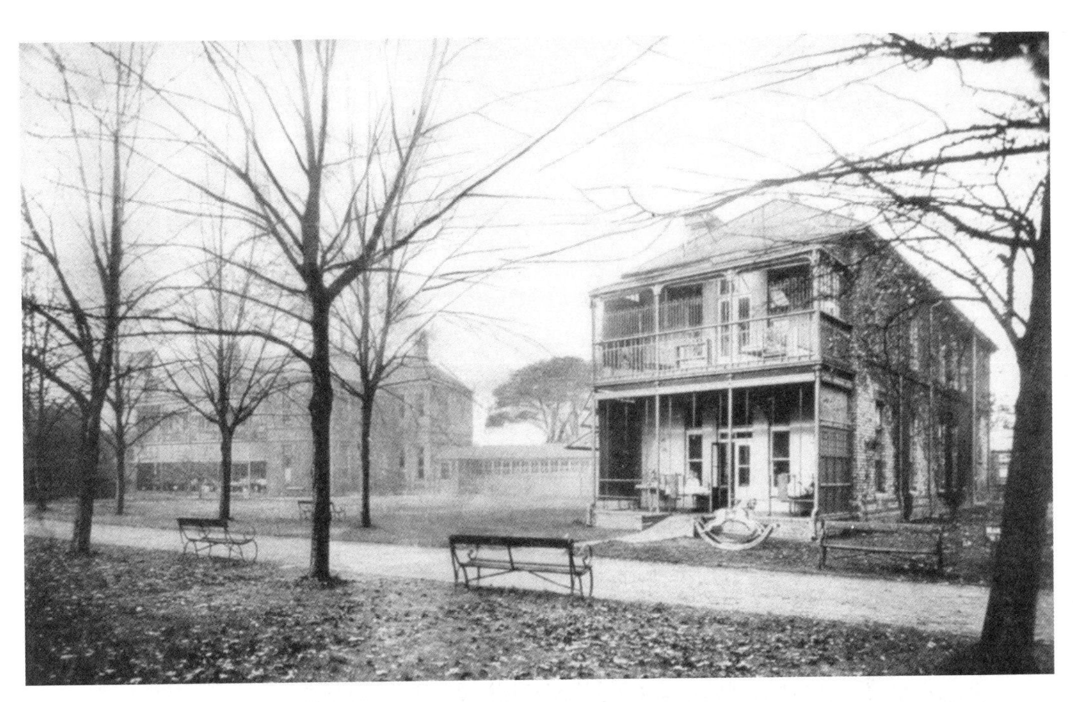

In the 1920s the hospital published a souvenir album, from which the next five pictures are taken. This one shows the grounds with the children's block in the foreground and Marlborough and Rowney wards to the left. Marlborough and Rowney were men's wards, completed in 1894.

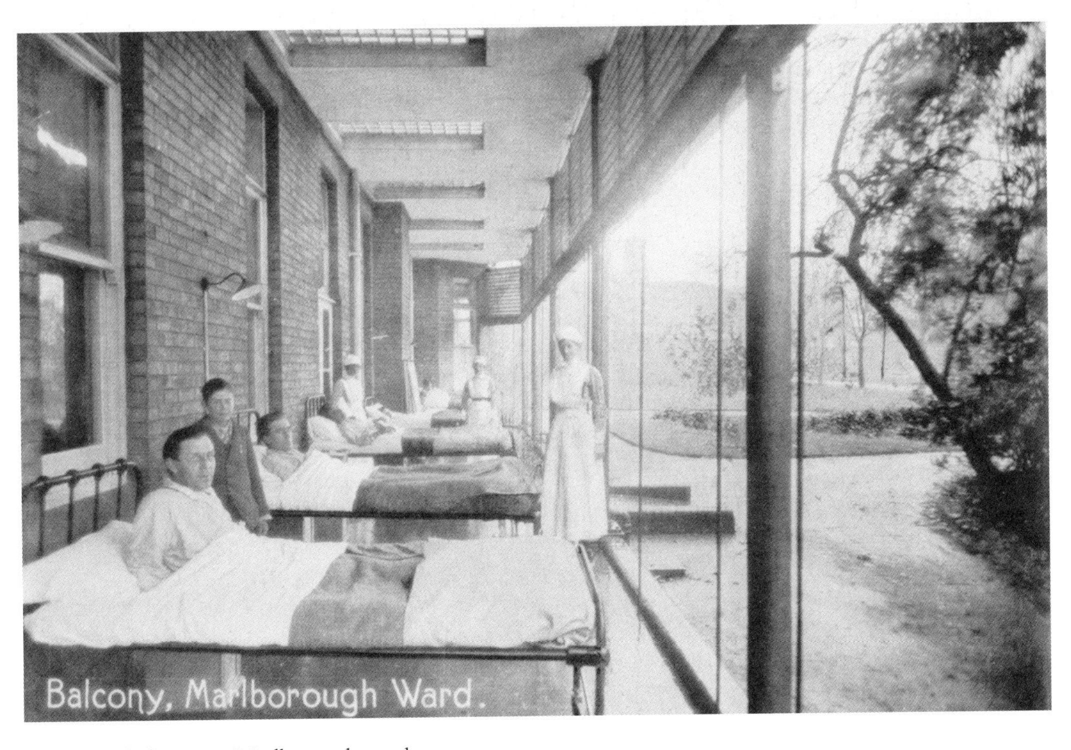

The balcony on Marlborough ward.

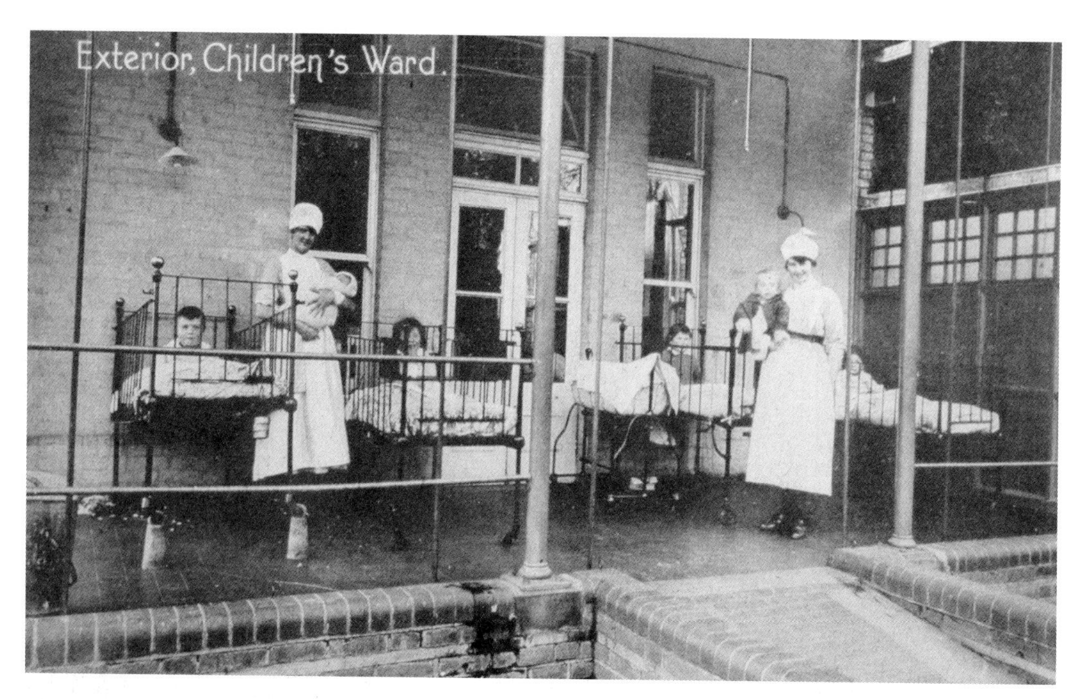

Nurses Fishlock and Jones tend patients from the children's ward. The building was extended and the balconies enclosed in 1937.

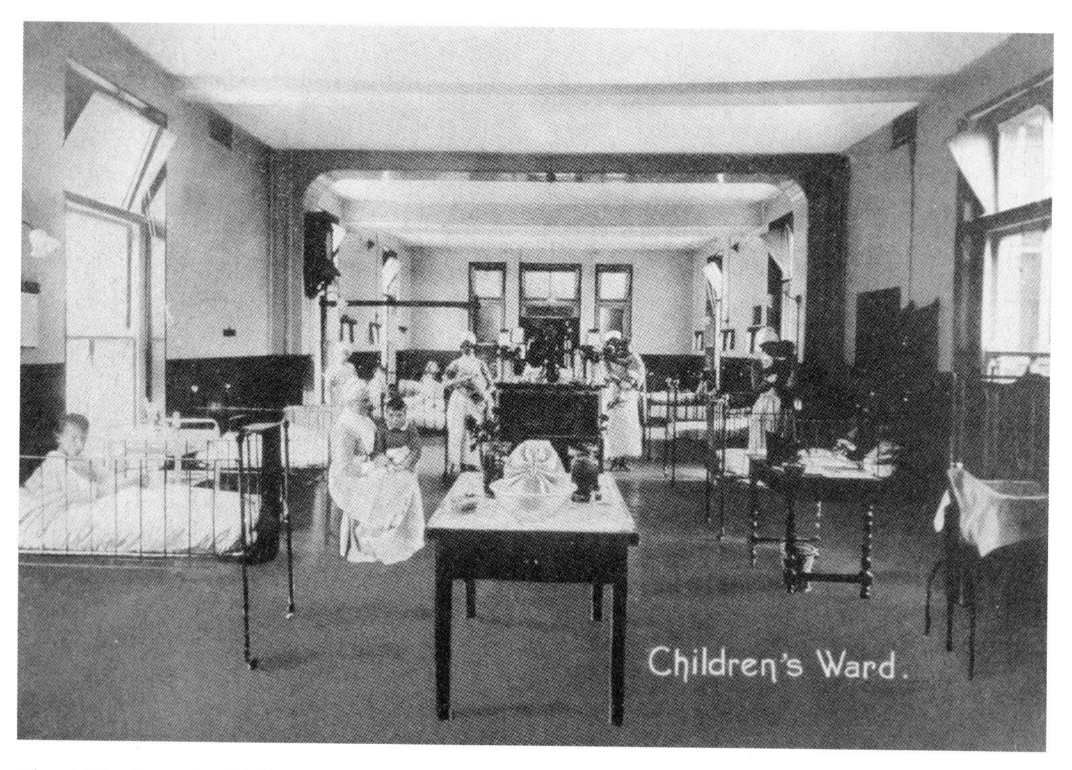

The children's ward, *c.* 1922.

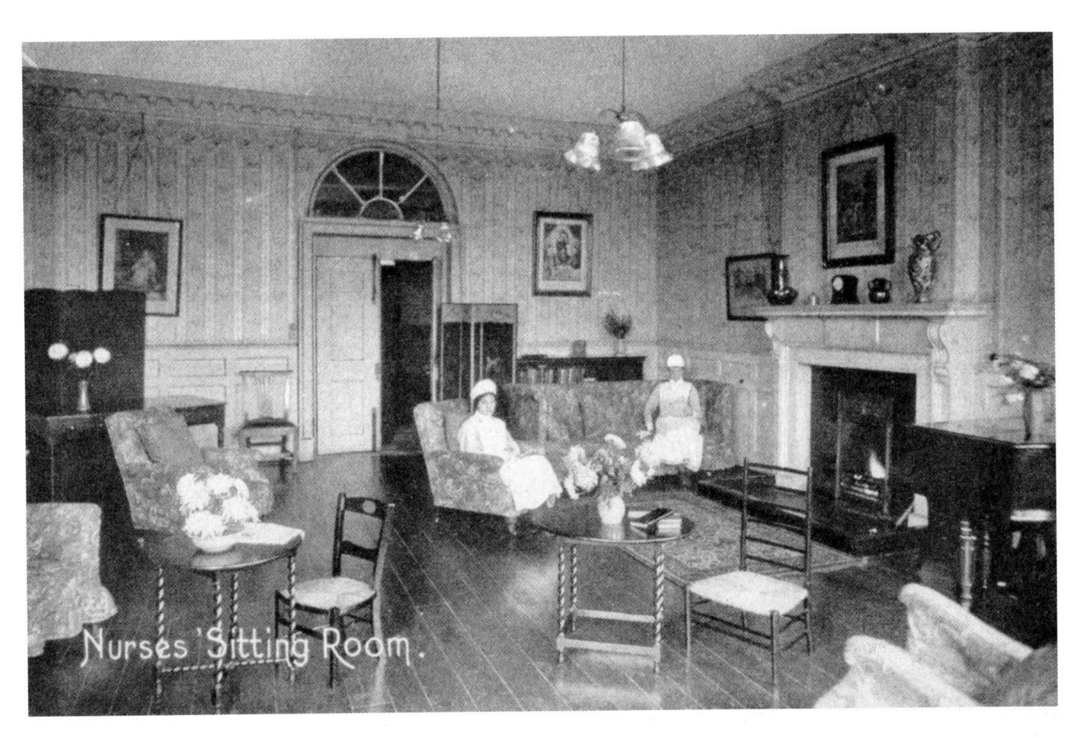

The nurses' sitting room, *c.* 1922.

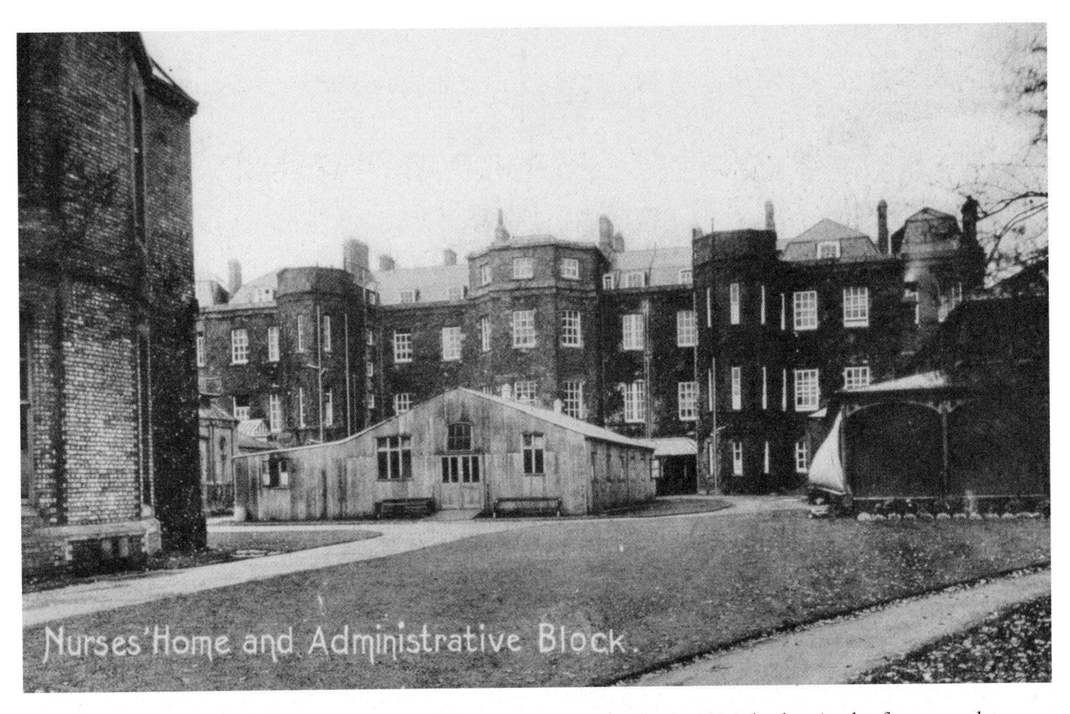

The administrative block (the original hospital) from the back, *c.* 1922. The hut in the foreground was a temporary outpatient department while the new buildings at the front (1913) were being built. It was used as a ward during the First World War, and then as a social centre for dances and entertainment.

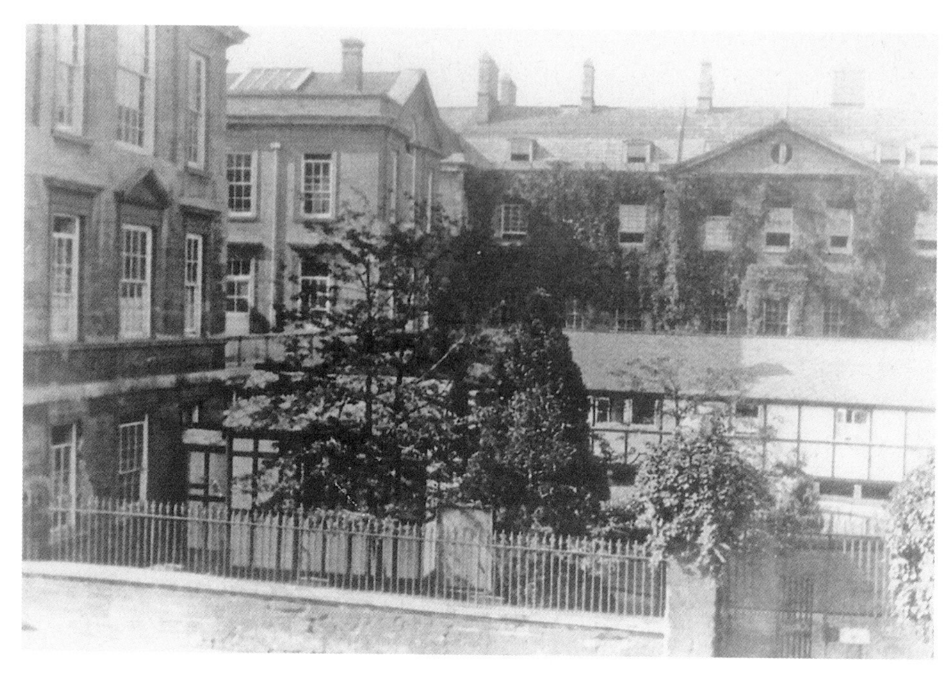

Although the hospital now owned the Manor House site, it was some years before developments began there and the Radcliffe trustees were still resisting approaches from the Infirmary to buy the Observatory. As a result, nurses had to live in these wooden huts in the forecourt, pictured around 1922.

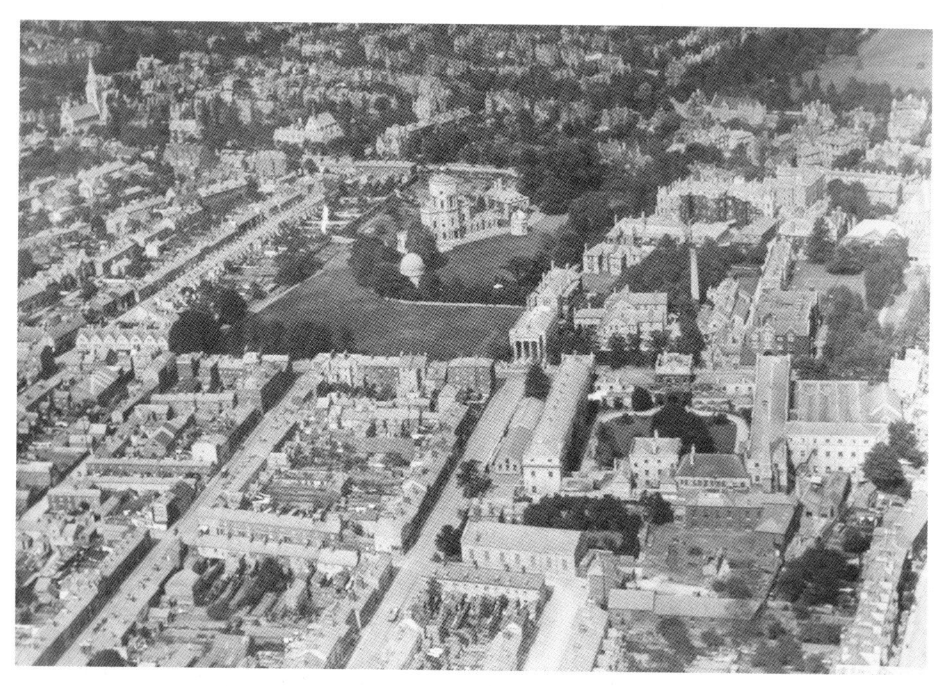

An aerial view of the site before the acquisition of the Observatory, *c.* 1929. St Paul's Church and the Eye Hospital are prominent centre right.

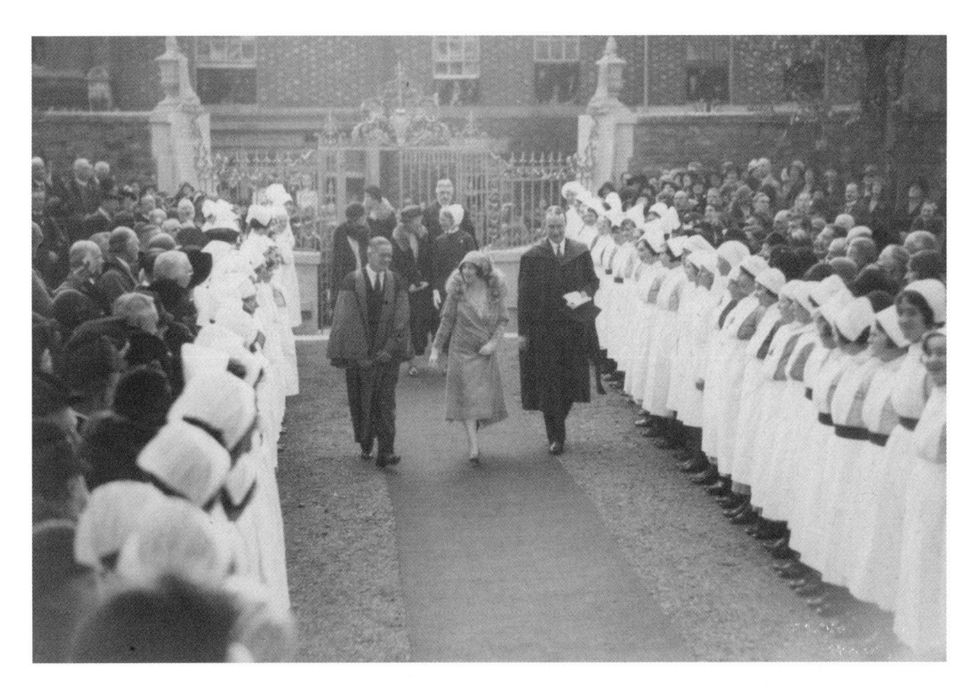

Relief came at the end of the decade when negotiations to buy the Observatory were at last successful, and Sir William Morris provided the money. It began a new era of expansion starting with the new maternity department which was opened by the Duchess of York (later the Queen and then Queen Mother) on 22 October 1931.

Sir William Morris (left) and the Duchess of York step out on the red carpet at the opening. Sir William provided £38,000 for the building.

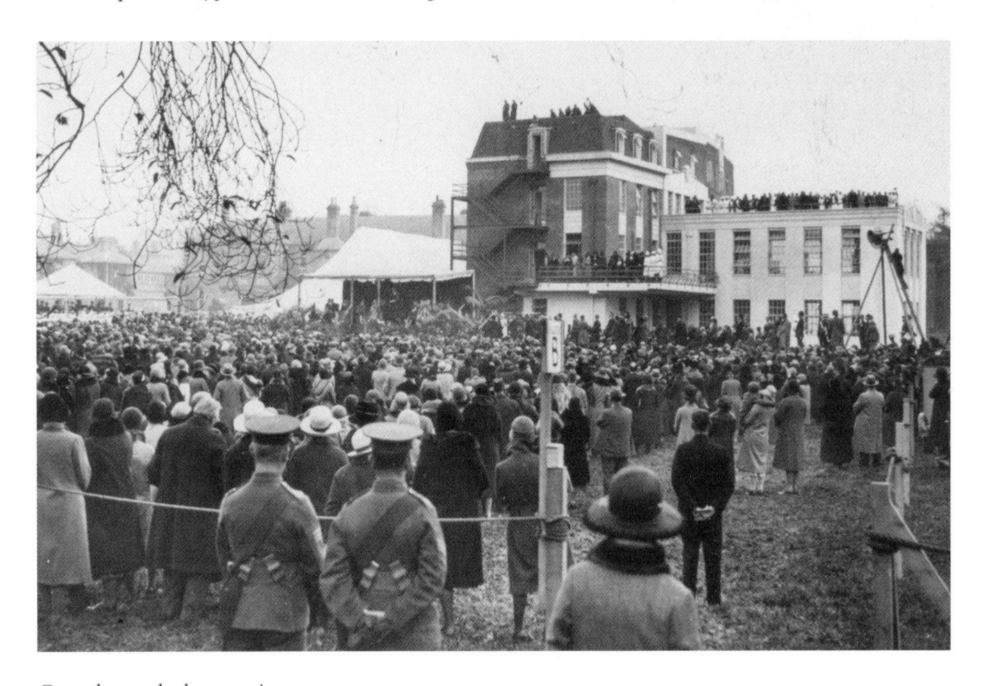

Crowds watch the opening ceremony.

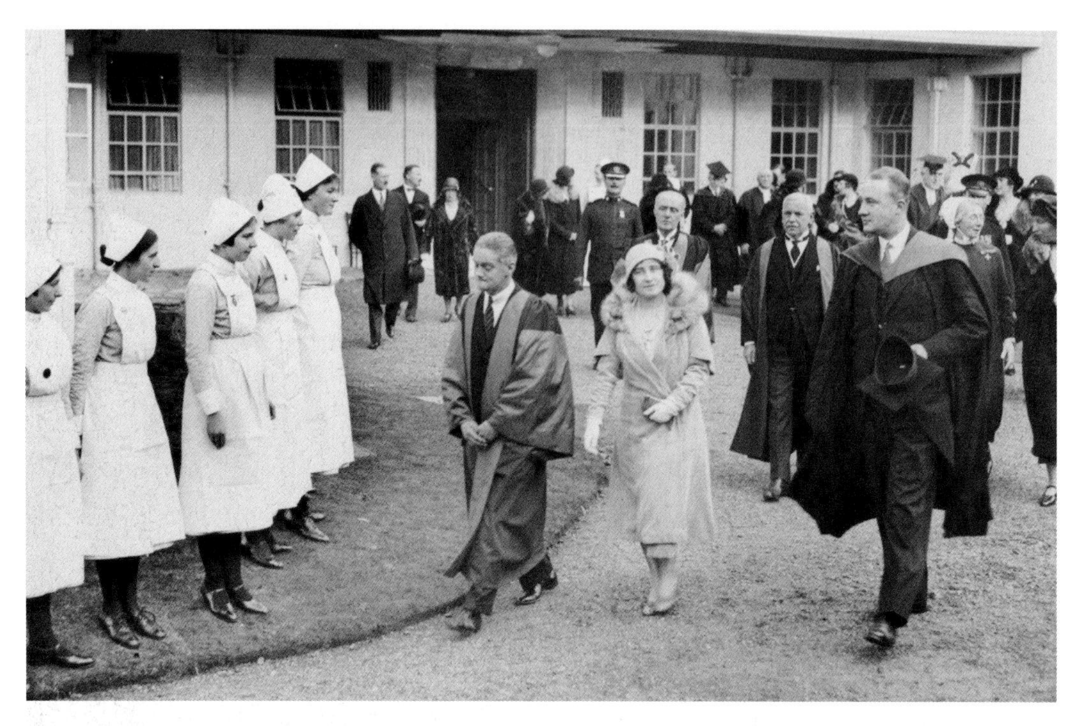

Sir William Morris strides ahead as the royal party leave the building.

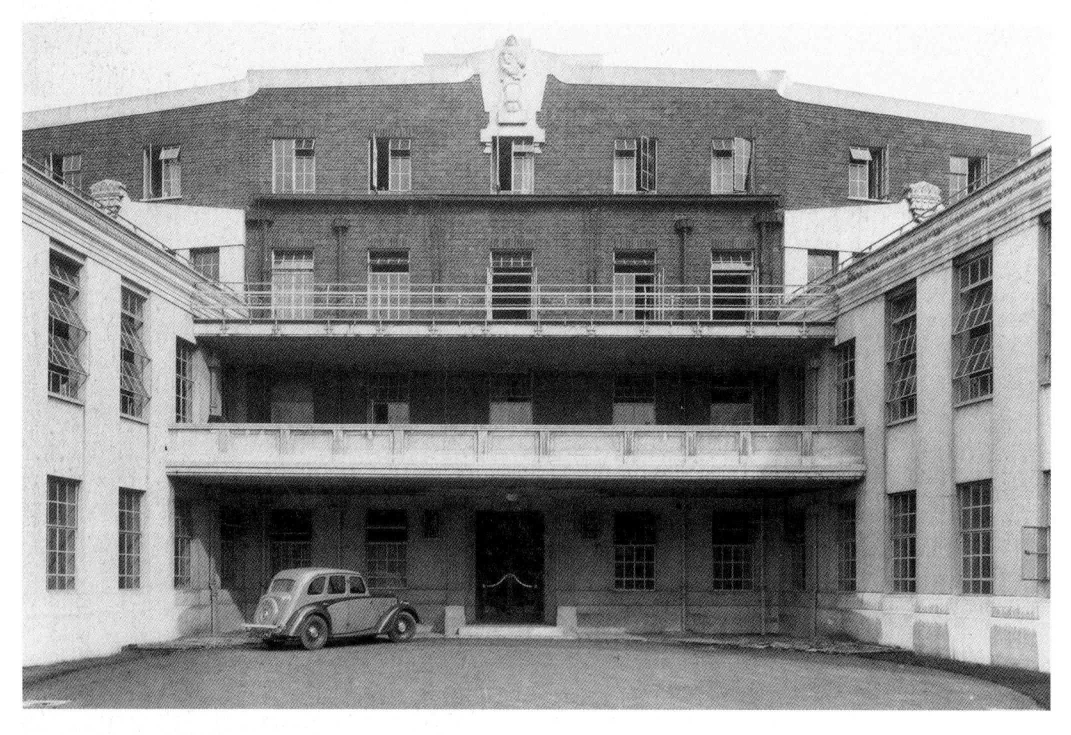

The Radcliffe Maternity Home (1931). Twenty-five years later the mother of the first baby born there unveiled a plaque to rename it the Nuffield Maternity Home.

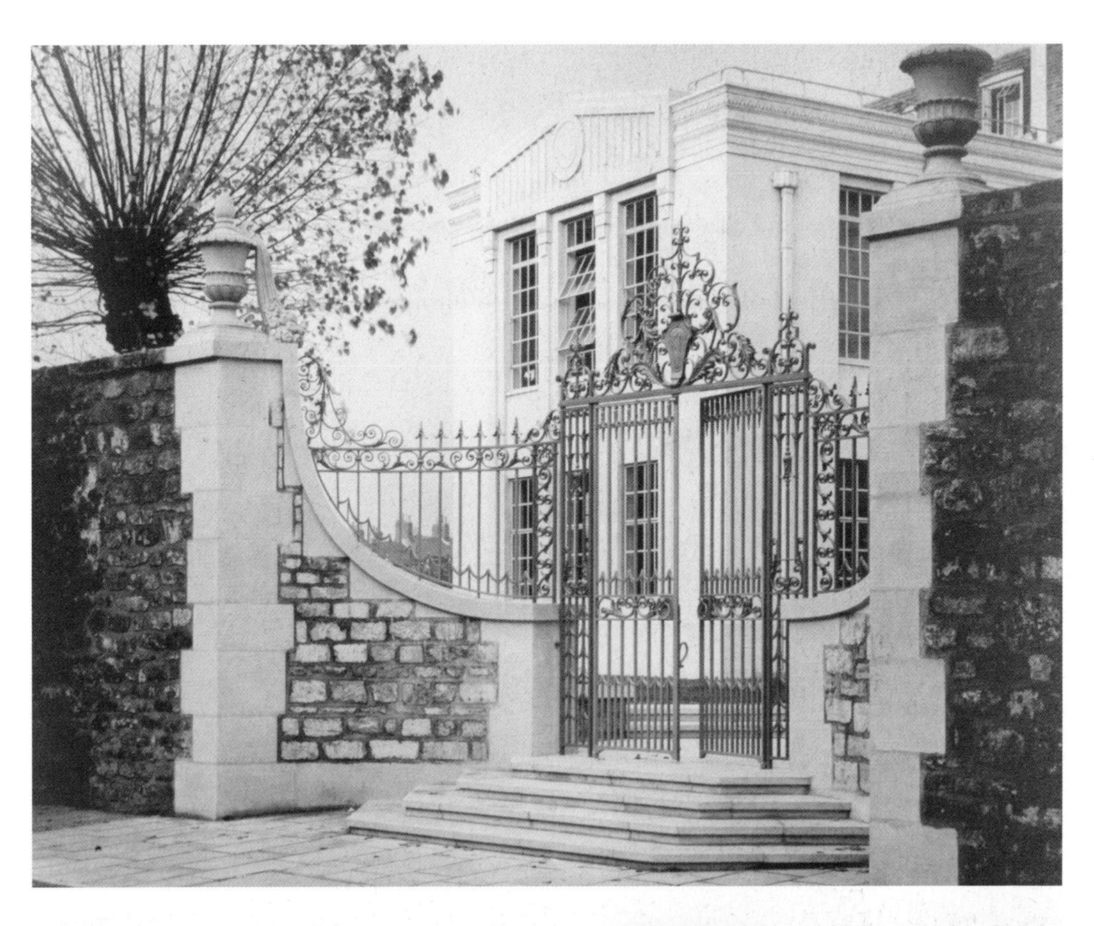

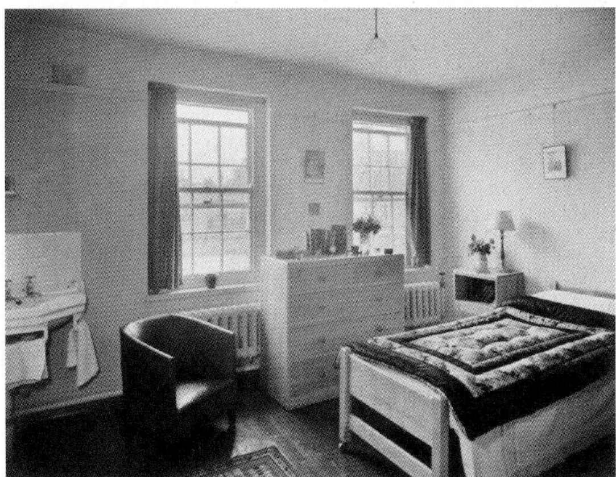

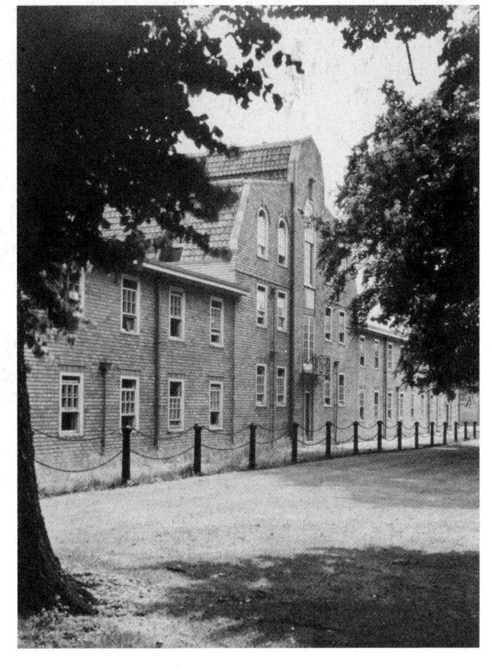

Top: The handsome gates of the maternity home.

Above: A nurse's bedroom, *c.* 1932.

Right: New wards and new departments followed, including a new nurses' home, pictured here around 1932.

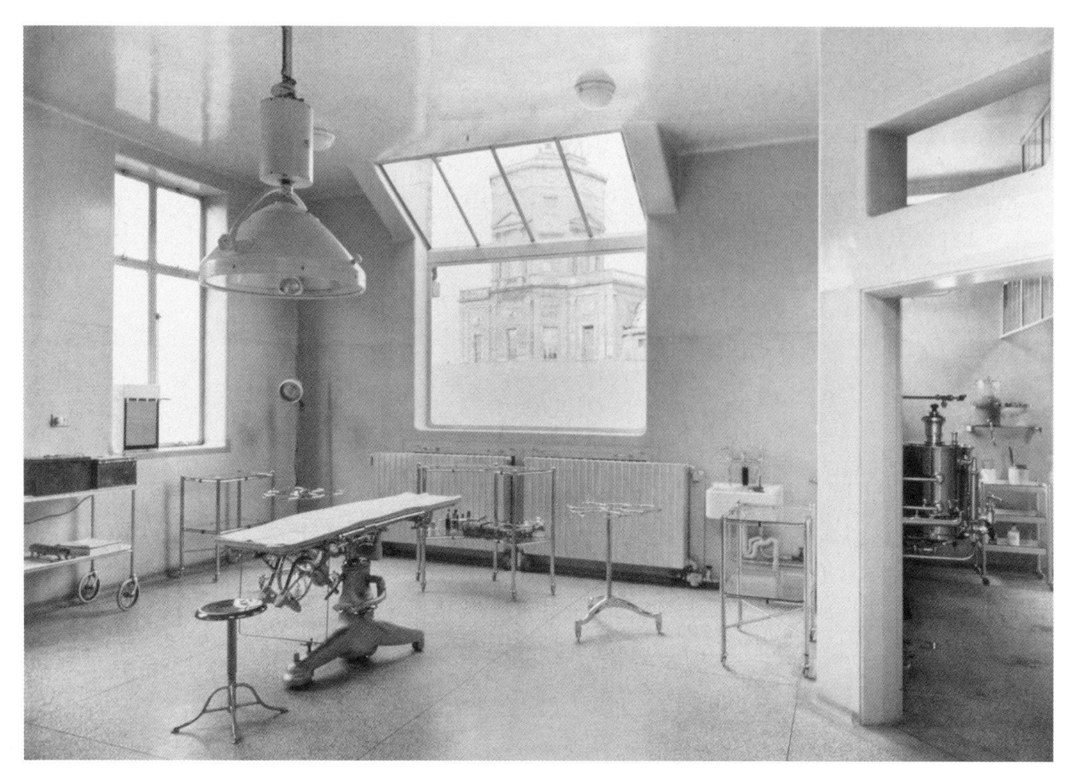

An operating theatre, *c.* 1938. This shows more modern equipment and a view of the Observatory tower through the window.

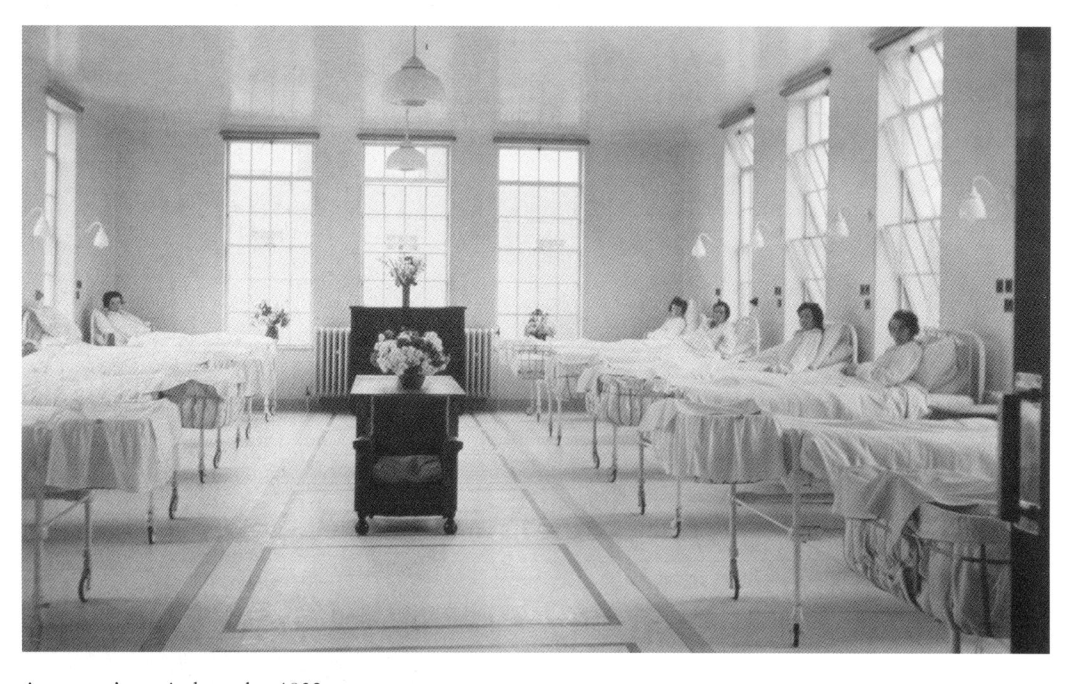

A women's surgical ward, *c.* 1932.

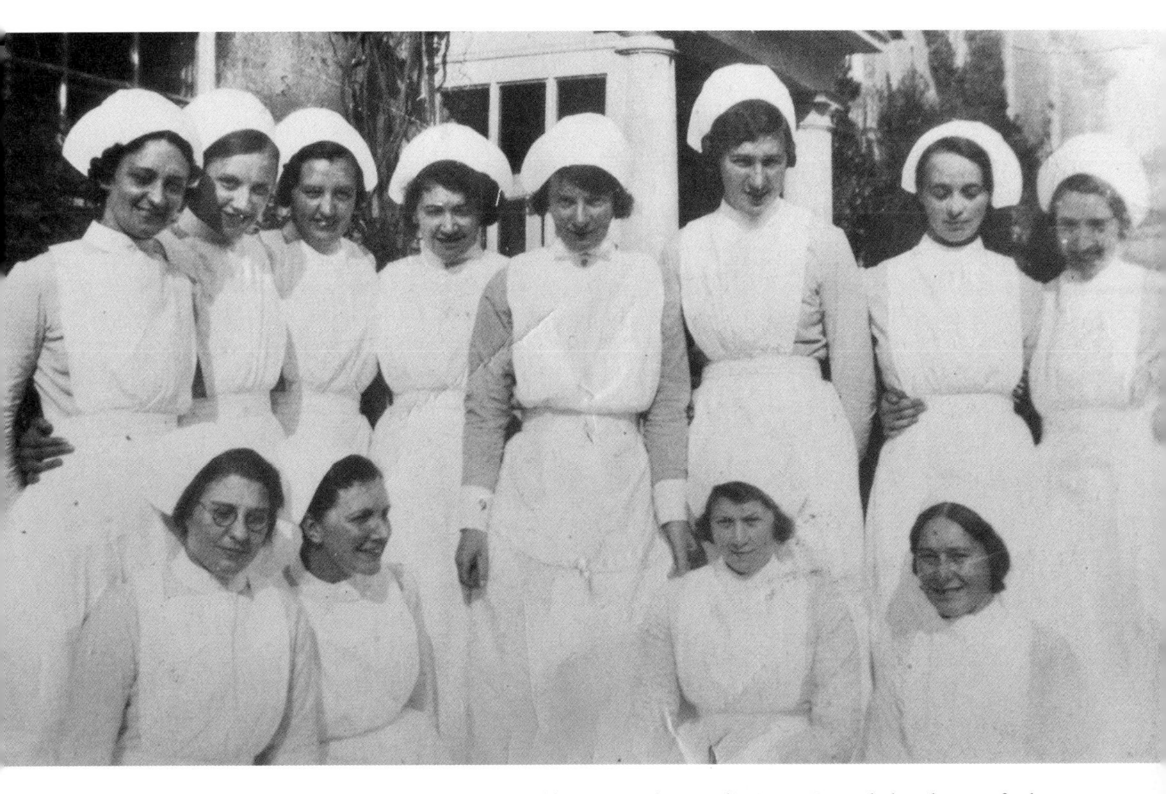

Above: Among the first to occupy the new nurses' home was the novelist Mary Renault, best known for her books about ancient Greece, who trained as a nurse in the early 1930s. Her real name was Mary Challans and after she left in 1936, she drew on her experiences in a novel, *Purposes of Love*, which explored a range of sexual relationships in what the *Sunday Pictorial* called, 'one of the frankest and most intimate love stories of recent years'.

It was at this time that the matron had chocks screwed to the windows of the nurses' home so that they would open only far enough to let in some air.

The book contains passages which derive from Mary's experience, describing the arduous routine, the tiredness and the pathos as a nineteen-year-old girl sits on a balcony beside a dying boy stitching the shroud he will soon wear.

This shows Mary Challans (Mary Renault) in the front row, second from left with fellow nurses in training, *c.* 1930-36.

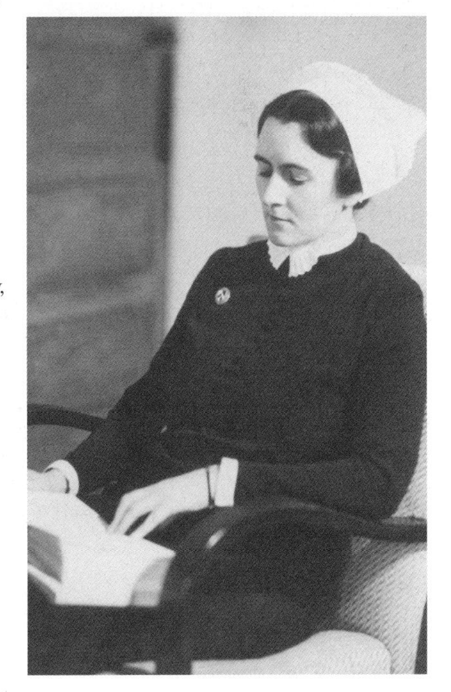

Right: Margaret Bonthron, matron from 1937 to 1942. Robb-Smith describes her as a woman of charm, selfless devotion and great ability, who had maintained a high standard of nursing care in two difficult periods – the opening of the new Nuffield Departments and the wartime disruption.

She took a strong interest in training. The year she retired there were 730 enquiries about nurse training and ninety-three candidates were accepted. Vacancies in the school were booked for a year ahead.

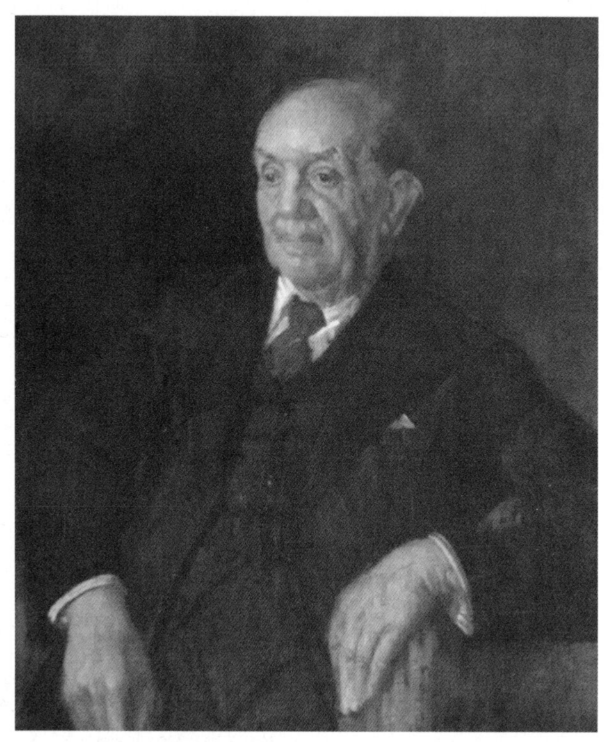

E. Cecil Bevers 1876-1962
He was surgeon to the Infirmary from 1904 to 1933. Short and stocky, he was regarded as the most able of all the surgeons at the time – a swift operator and a popular teacher.

He had a severe squint and it was said that nobody quite knew which eye was on the surgery or where the other one was looking. He retired to Devon in 1933 but returned in 1938 and immediately became chairman of the management committee. From 1942 to 1946, when the surgical staff was depleted, he resumed active surgery. In tandem with the administrator Arthur Sanctuary, he carried the hospital through the war years and the transition to the NHS when he became the first chairman of governors of United Oxford Hospitals in 1948.

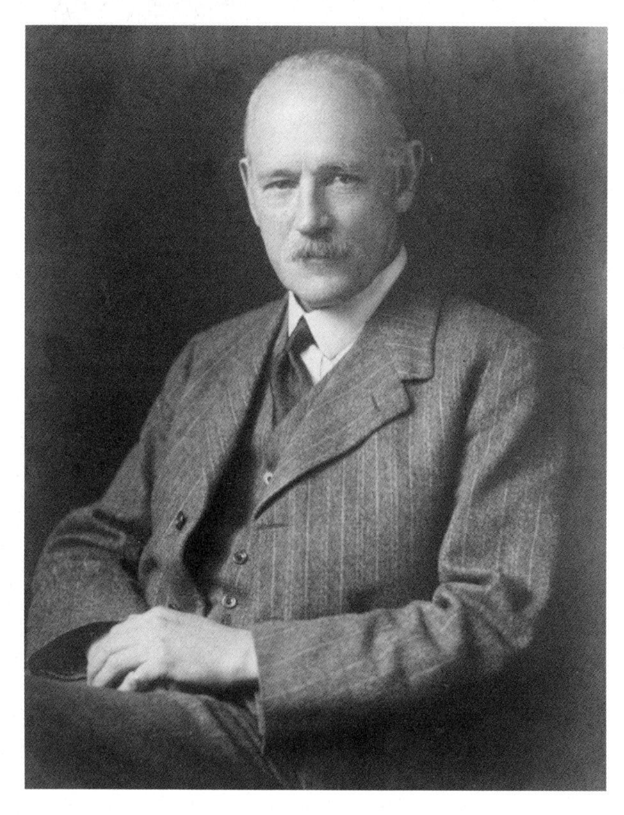

Sir Farquhar Buzzard 1871-1945
Appointed Regius Professor of Medicine in 1928, he had been an outstanding sportsman at Oxford and later played for the Old Carthusian team which won the FA Amateur Cup in 1892 and 1897. He was an ally of innovation and reform and played golf at Huntercombe, where he had the ear of Lord Nuffield with whose generous support he advanced the Oxford Medical School and established the first Nuffield departments. He foresaw the coming of the NHS and the end of the voluntary era and used his influence and position to make change more palatable to some of his colleagues. Robb-Smith describes him as, 'one of the greatest medical statesmen of his time.'

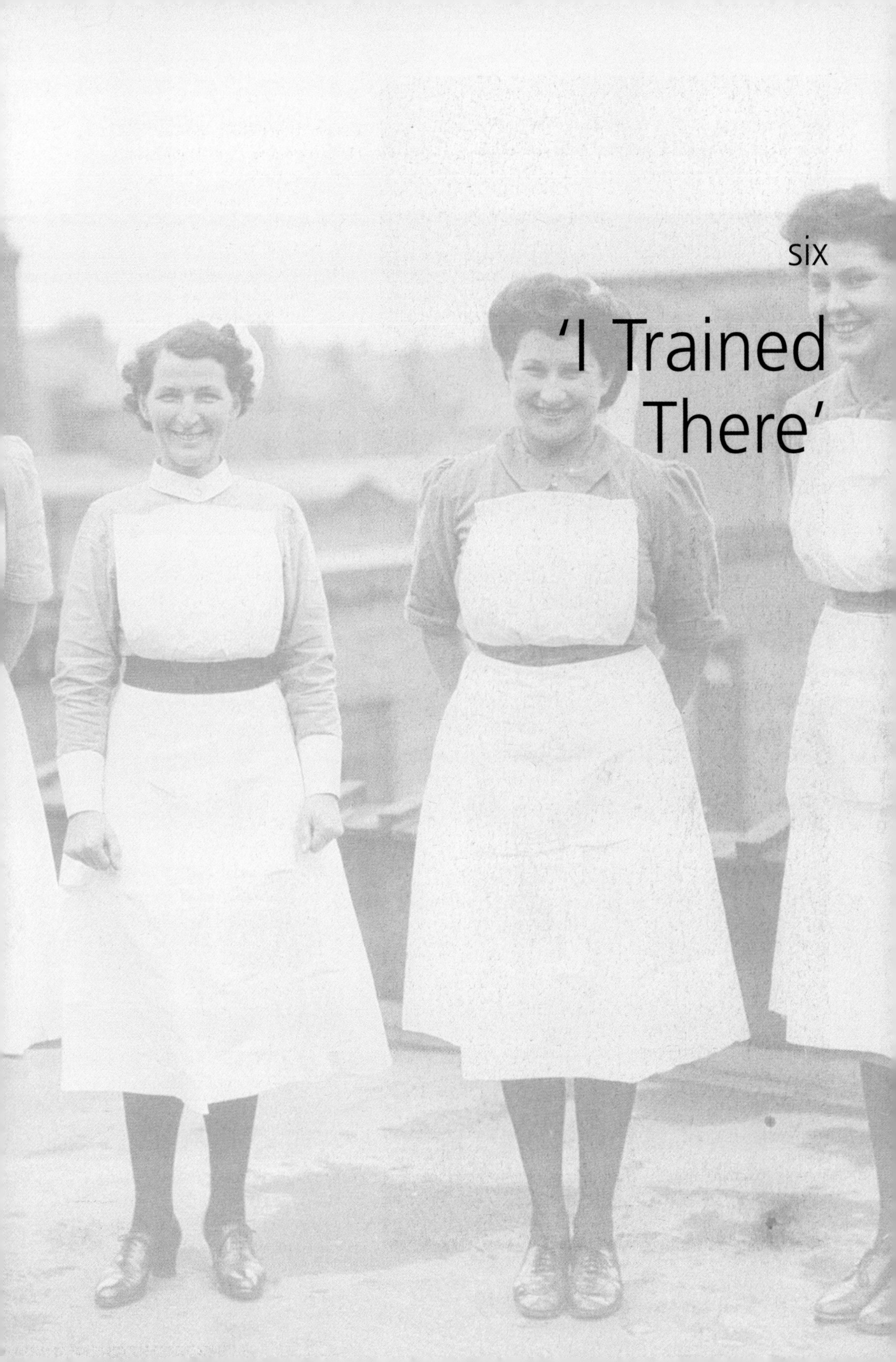

six

'I Trained There'

Many nurses who trained and worked at the Infirmary retain a strong affection for the hospital and keep in contact through the Radcliffe Guild of Nurses whose members meet for regular reunions.

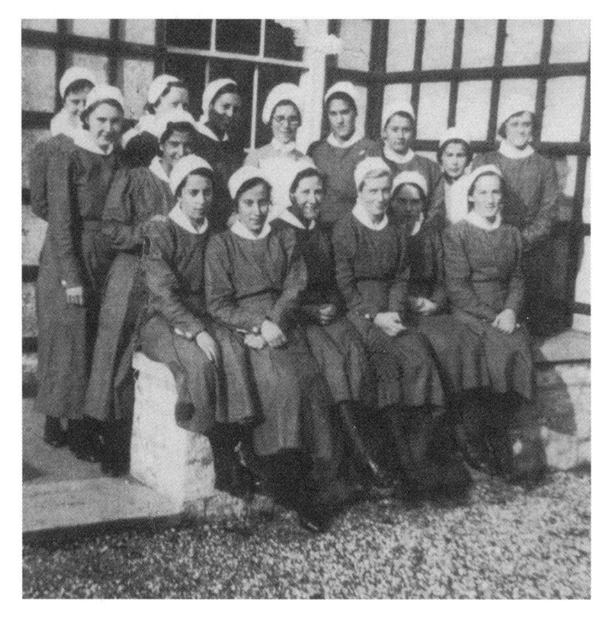

The Preliminary Training School intake for nurse training in 1938, loaned by Mrs Minnie Pritchard (*née* Herbert) who is among the group which also includes two Smiths, and nurses French, Lavender, Carmana, Nandi, Pace, Johnson, Norris, Pritchard, Herbert, Rayon Jones and Wilson. In 1942 Minnie won the third year prize.

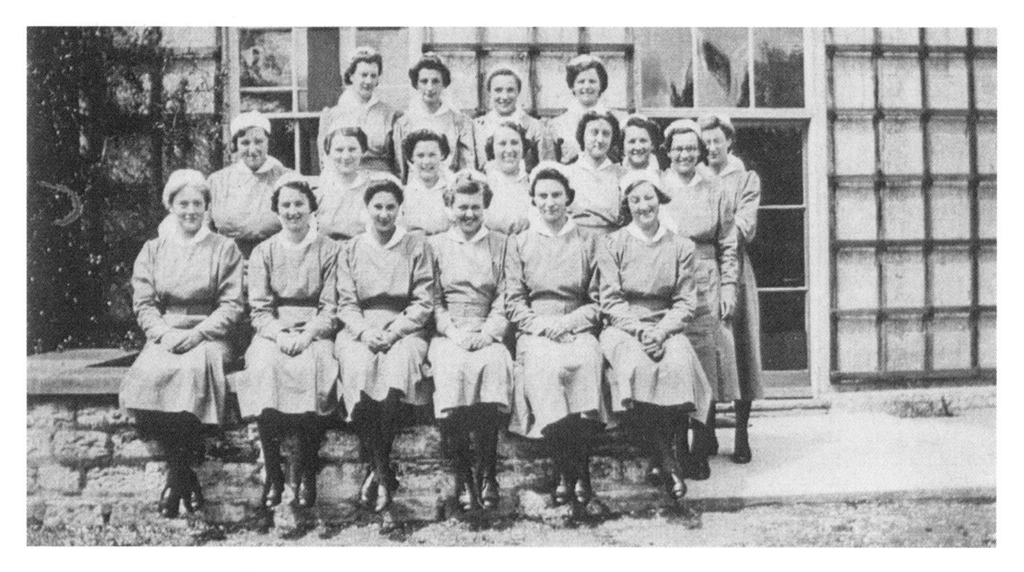

The May 1942 intake pictured at the Manor House. Sheila Brownlow, *née* Barnett (third from left, front row), recalls the strict but kind teaching of Sister Baldock. 'There was also a nurses' home off the side entrance to the Radcliffe', she writes. 'We used to climb over the bike sheds to get in on illicit late nights.'

From left to right, back row: -?-, Morecroft, Pyke, Jarman. Middle: Hampson, Price, Drew, Silver, Hodgson, Bex, Sullivan, Barnes. Front: Phelps, Dugdale, Barnett, Ryan, Slater, Plowden.

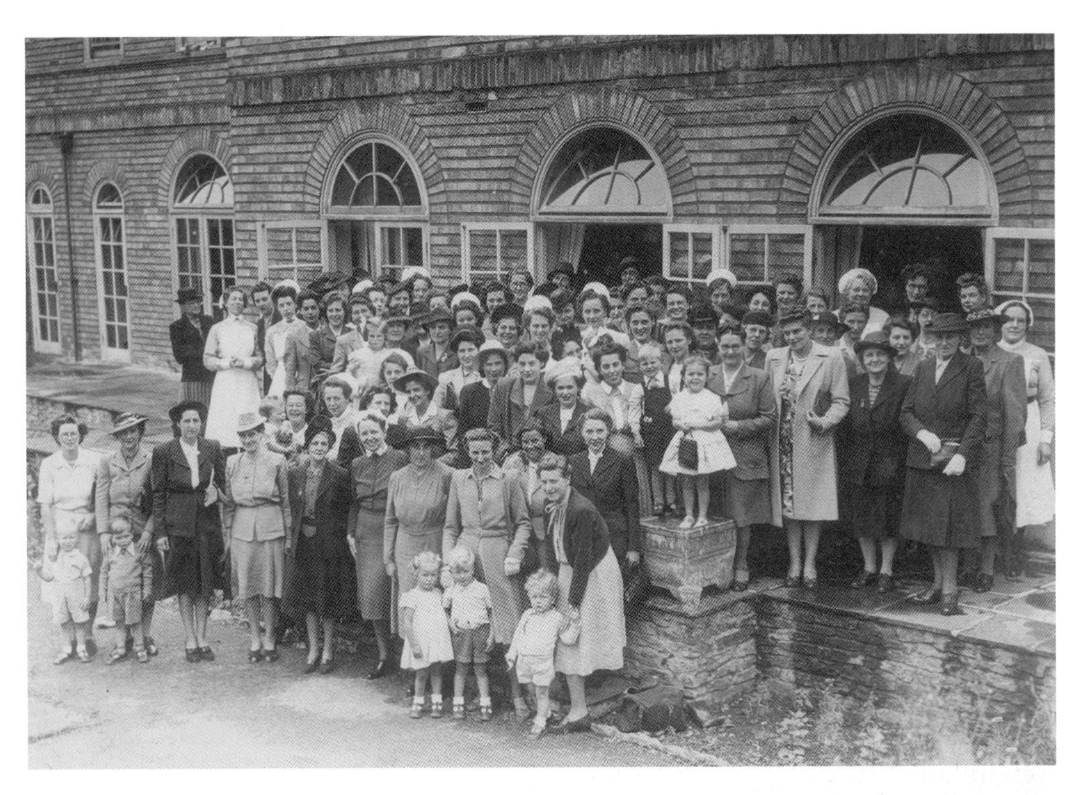

Reunion gatherings in 1947 (above) and 1949 (below).

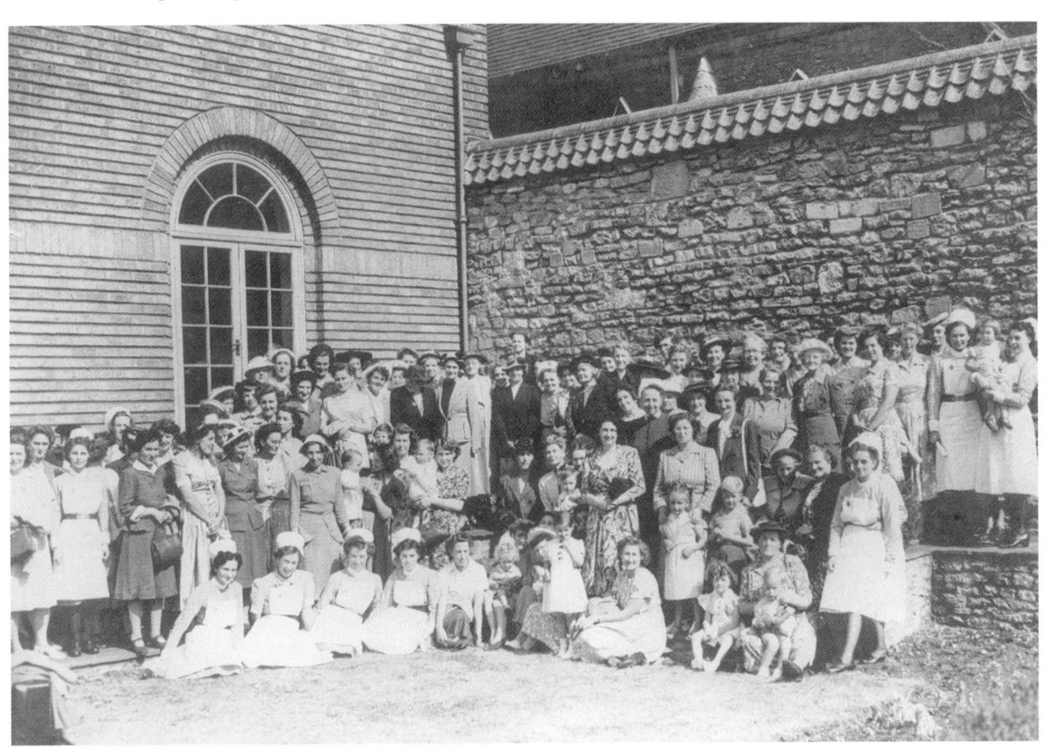

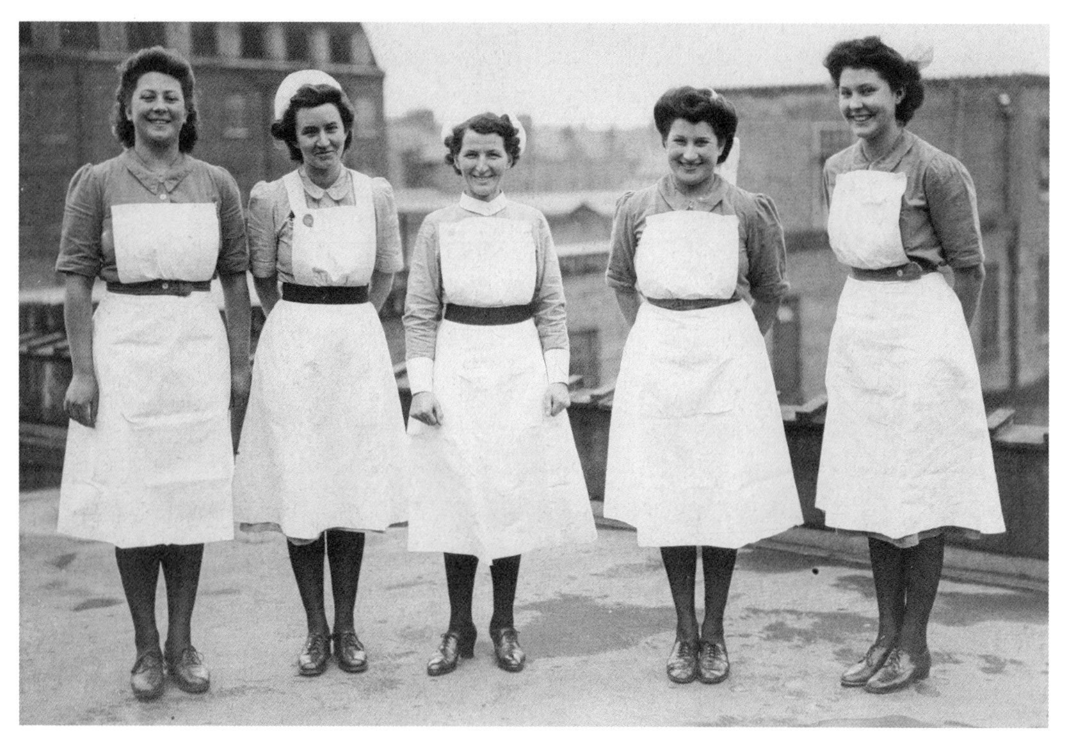

Symonds ward nurses on the roof in 1946. From left to right: Beryl Heaume, Charge Nurse Dugdale, Sister Virtue Wells, Betty Phillips (now Betty King, who sent the picture) and Dorothy Hickson.

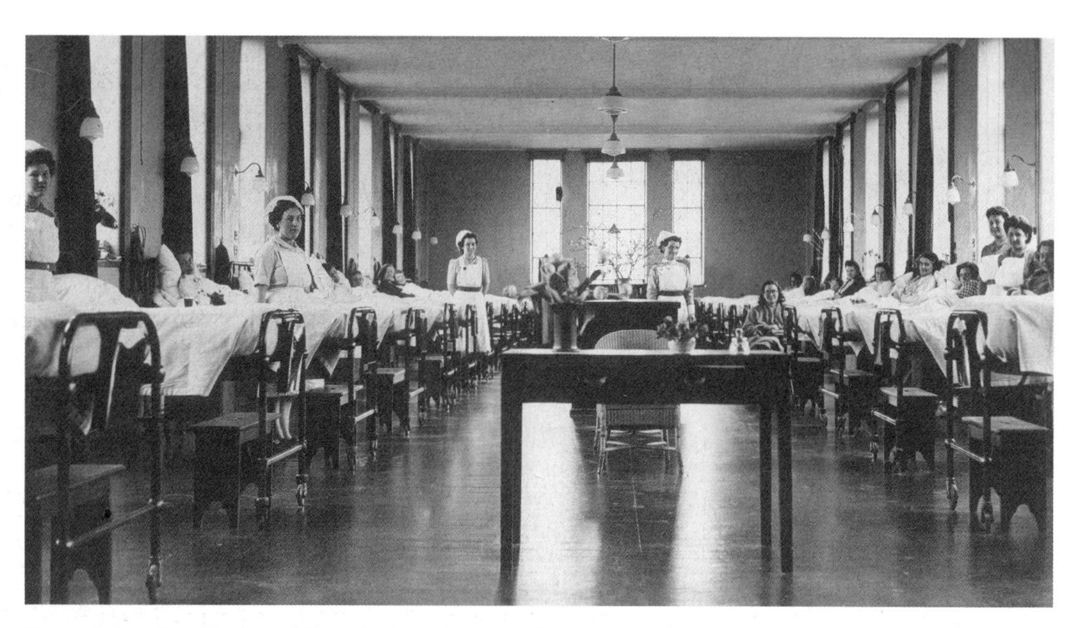

Symonds female surgical ward in 1946. Betty King recalls how seats under each bed had to be in line, bed wheels pointing the same way, ends of pillows facing away from the door and hospital corners on sheets and bedspreads. Sister Wells held a weekly service and served lunches from a heated trolley, which the nurses took to each patient.

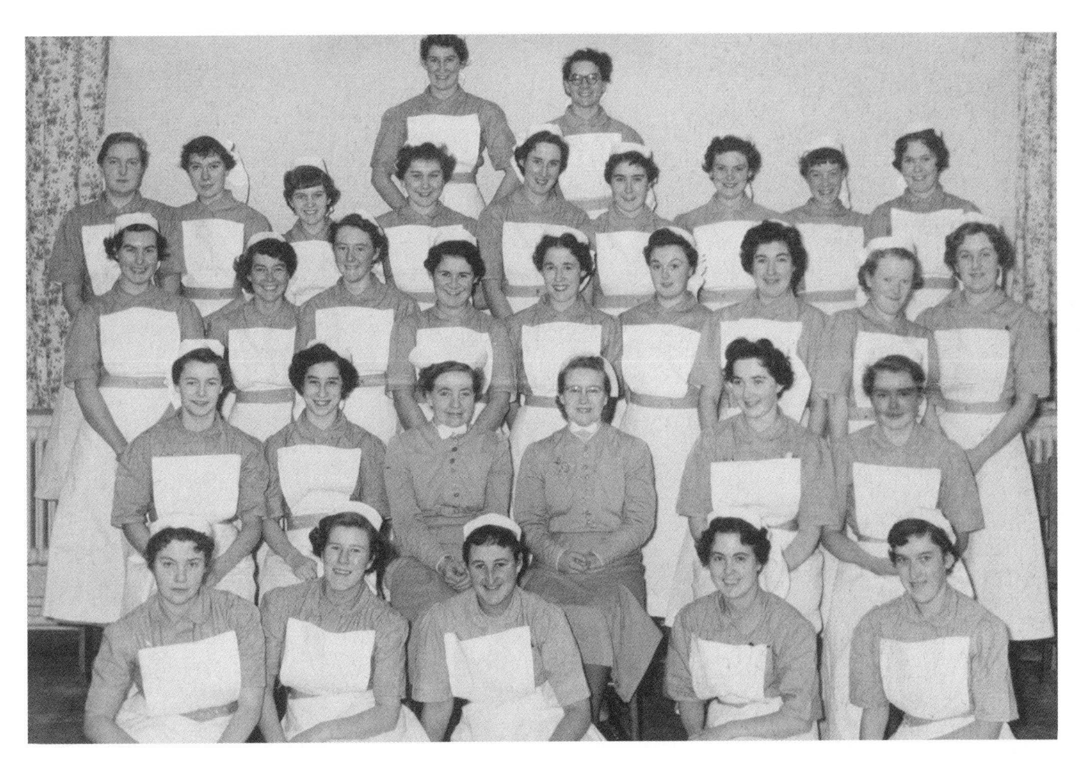

The October 1955 set of nurses starting their training.

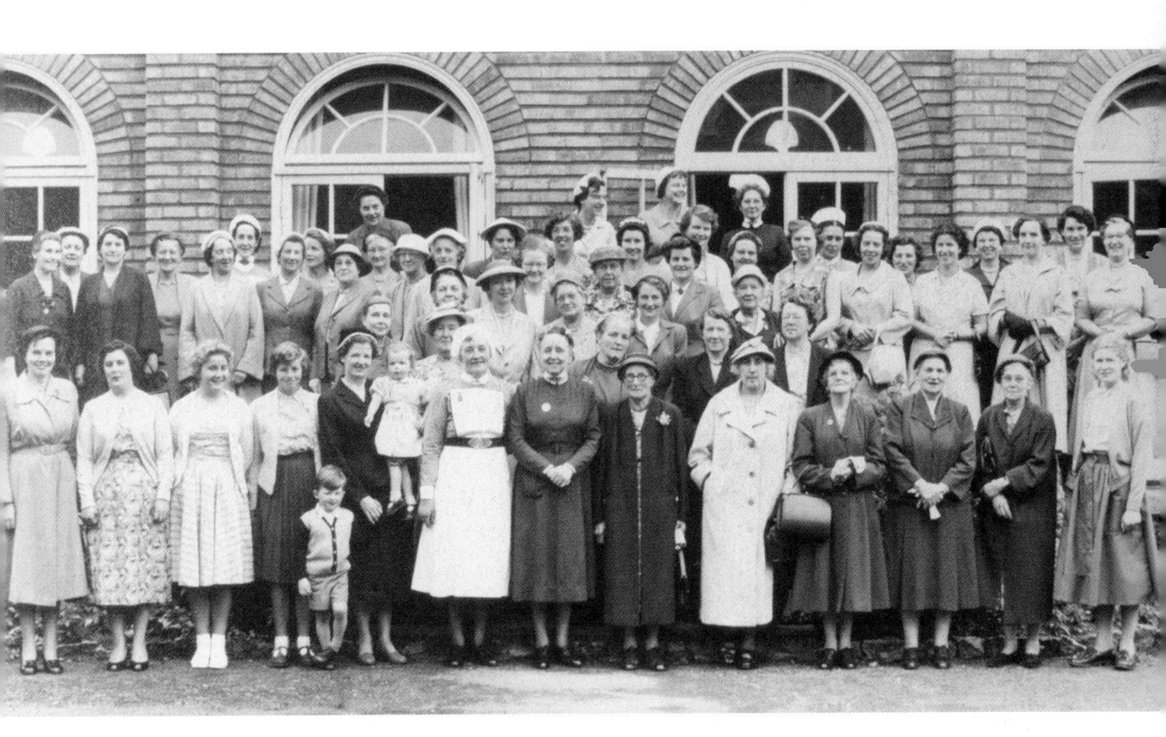

A reunion, *c.* 1958. Matron Edith Preddy (centre) joins current and former staff.

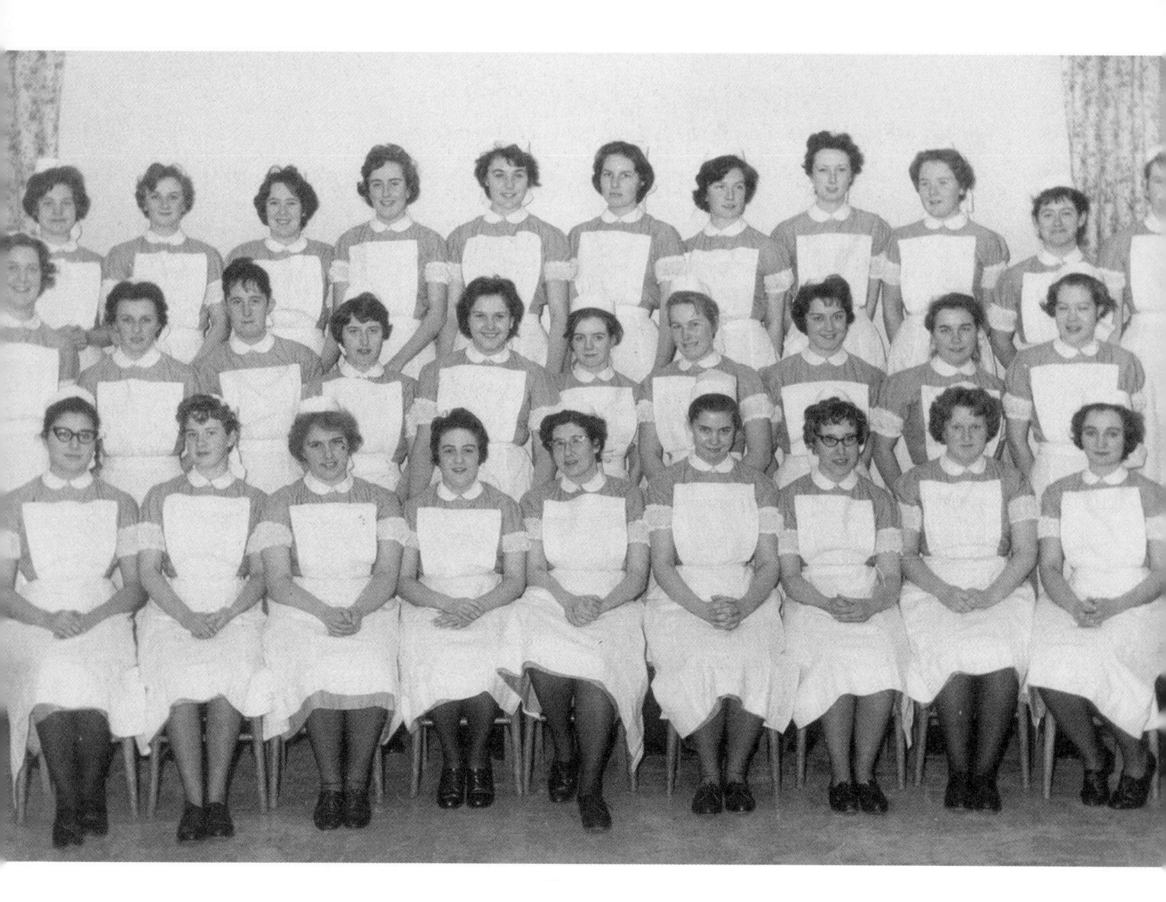

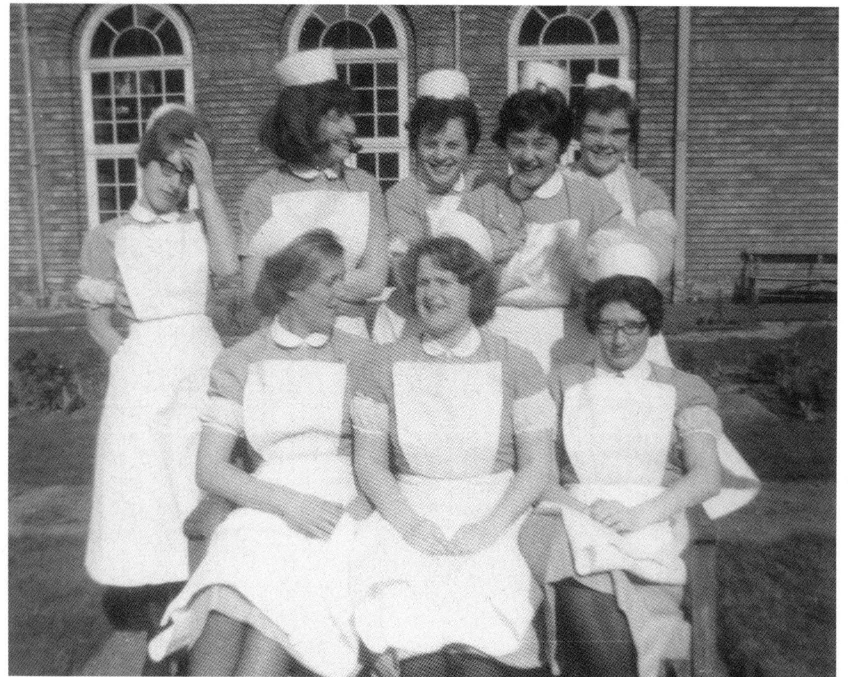

Above: The January 1962 set.

Left: A group from the January 1962 set sent in by Norma McMahon (front right) who writes, 'I have such happy memories of my Radcliffe days.' From left to right, back row: Janice Randal, Floss McGowan, Brenda Purnell, Margaret Bannister, Dorothy Garnett. Sitting: Elizabeth Wylie, Rosemary Jay, Norma McMahon.

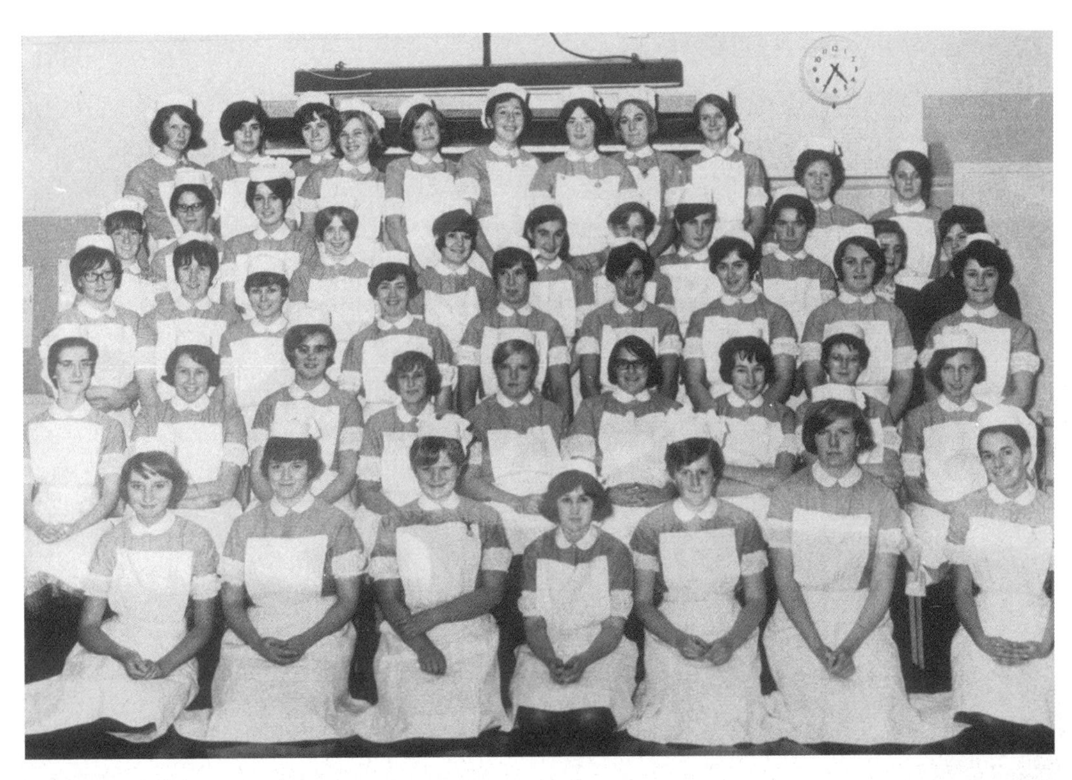

Above: The 1966 intake.

Below: The 1966 intake at a reunion thirty years after they began training together.

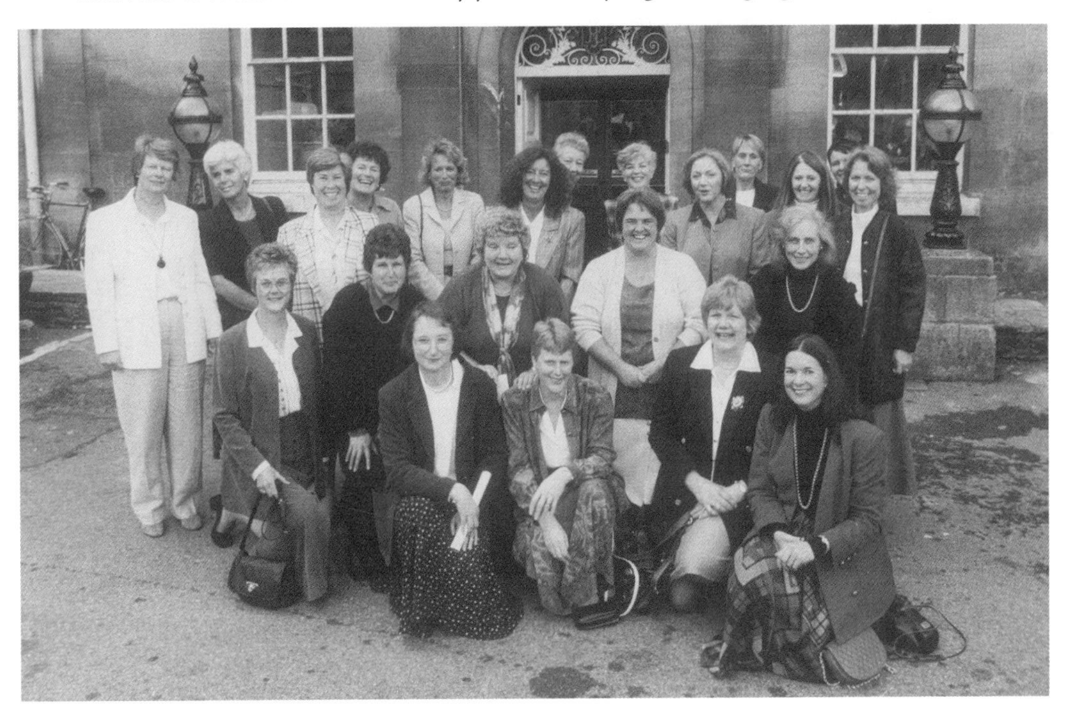

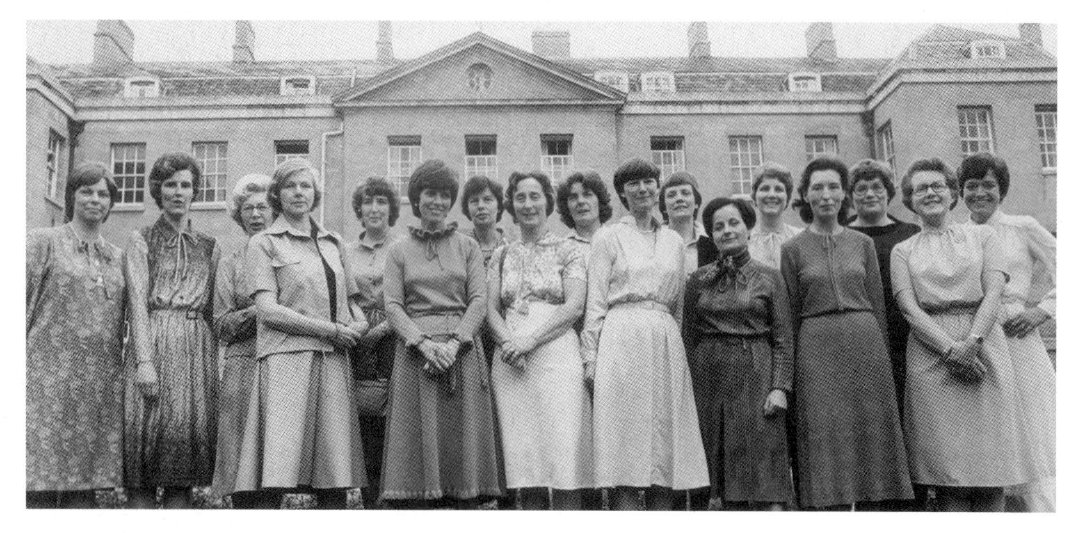

A 1981 reunion. From left to right: Joy Miller, Pat Aston, Anne Harold (Tutor), Di Smith, Mary Comley, Paddie McDonnell, Ann Brown, Molly Hadley, Julie Bailey, Pru Oswin, Rita Reed, Gaby Nadau, Claire Ryder, Alm Charles, Anne Footner, Sue Souch, Viv Wightman.

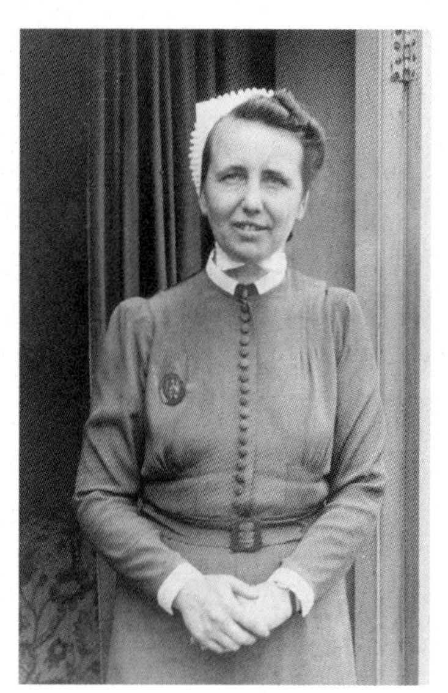

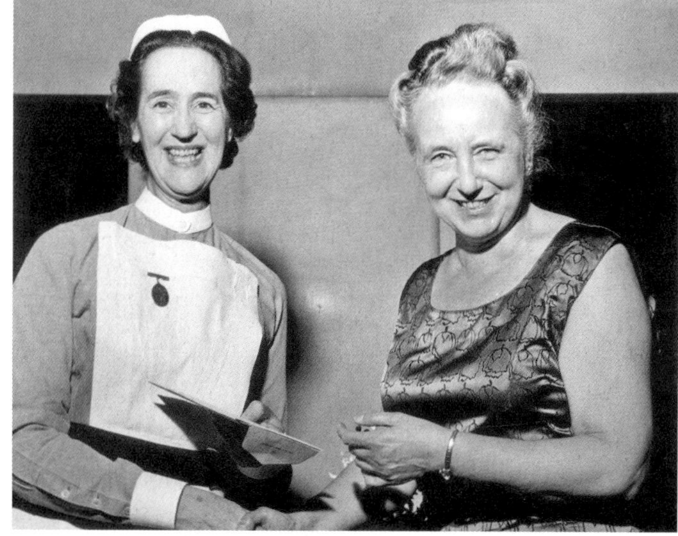

Above left: Edith Preddy, matron from 1942 to 1965. She was born in Bristol, trained at St Mary's Hospital, Paddington and worked in London, Hull and Leeds before moving to Oxford. Administrator E.J.R Burrough said she was, 'cast in the mould of authoritative and dedicated matrons'. She was said to dislike calling the junction of corridors 'Piccadilly' because it lowered the tone, but she was also the force behind the celebrated matron's ball which took place before Christmas each year. In 1949 she introduced a study day one day a week for student nurses. (*Oxford Mail and Times*)

Above right: More than 300 staff attended Miss Preddy's retirement party. During her time at the Radcliffe Infirmary the NHS had arrived, 231 beds had been added, nursing staff had doubled and medical staff trebled. In the picture Sister A.D. Day is making a presentation on behalf of the nurses.(*Oxford Mail and Times*)

seven

Life at the Radcliffe – 1

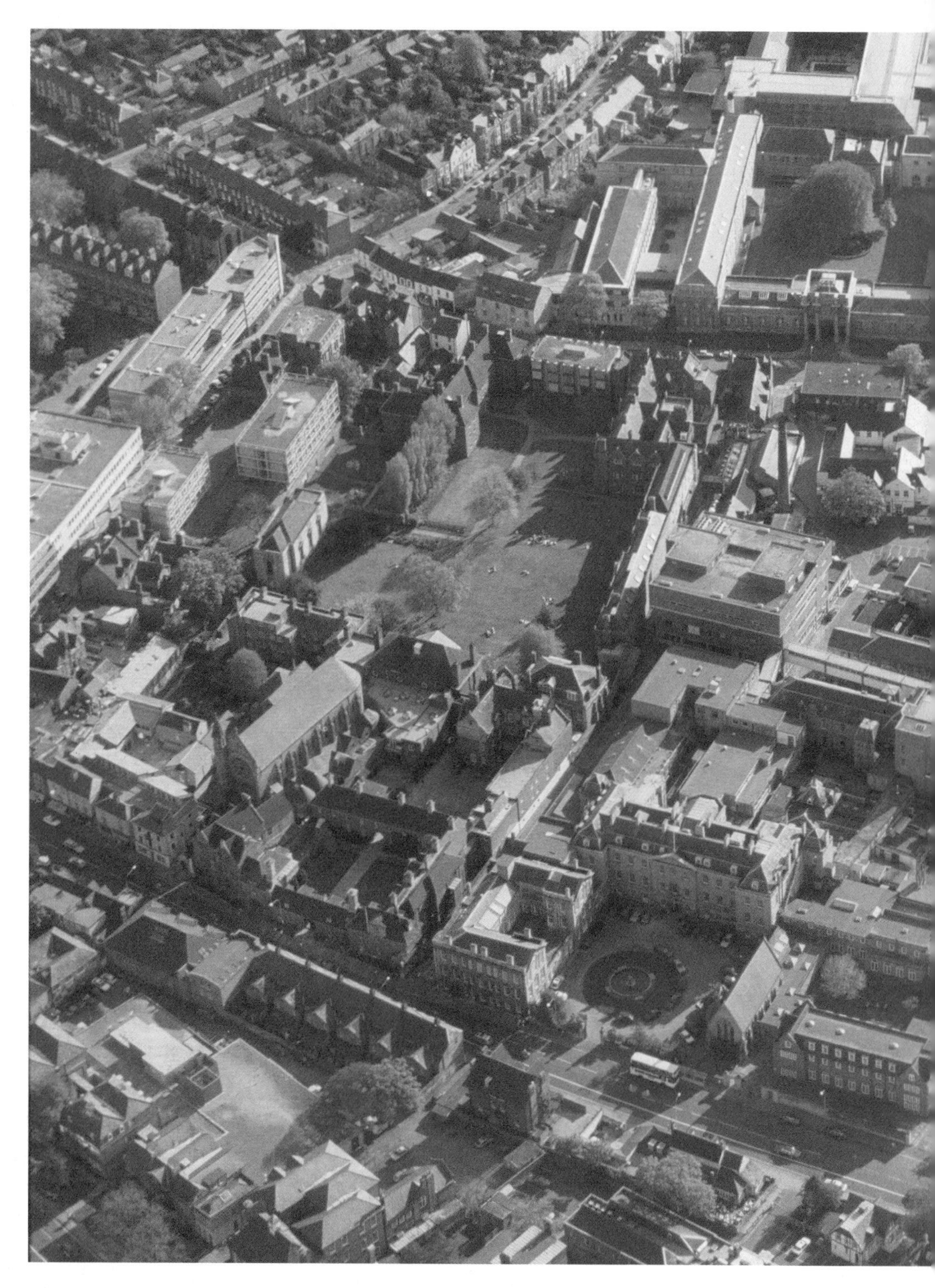

The Radcliffe from the air, *c.* 1975. The picture shows clearly how the Infirmary has wrapped itself around the Observatory with the major developments of the post-war period.

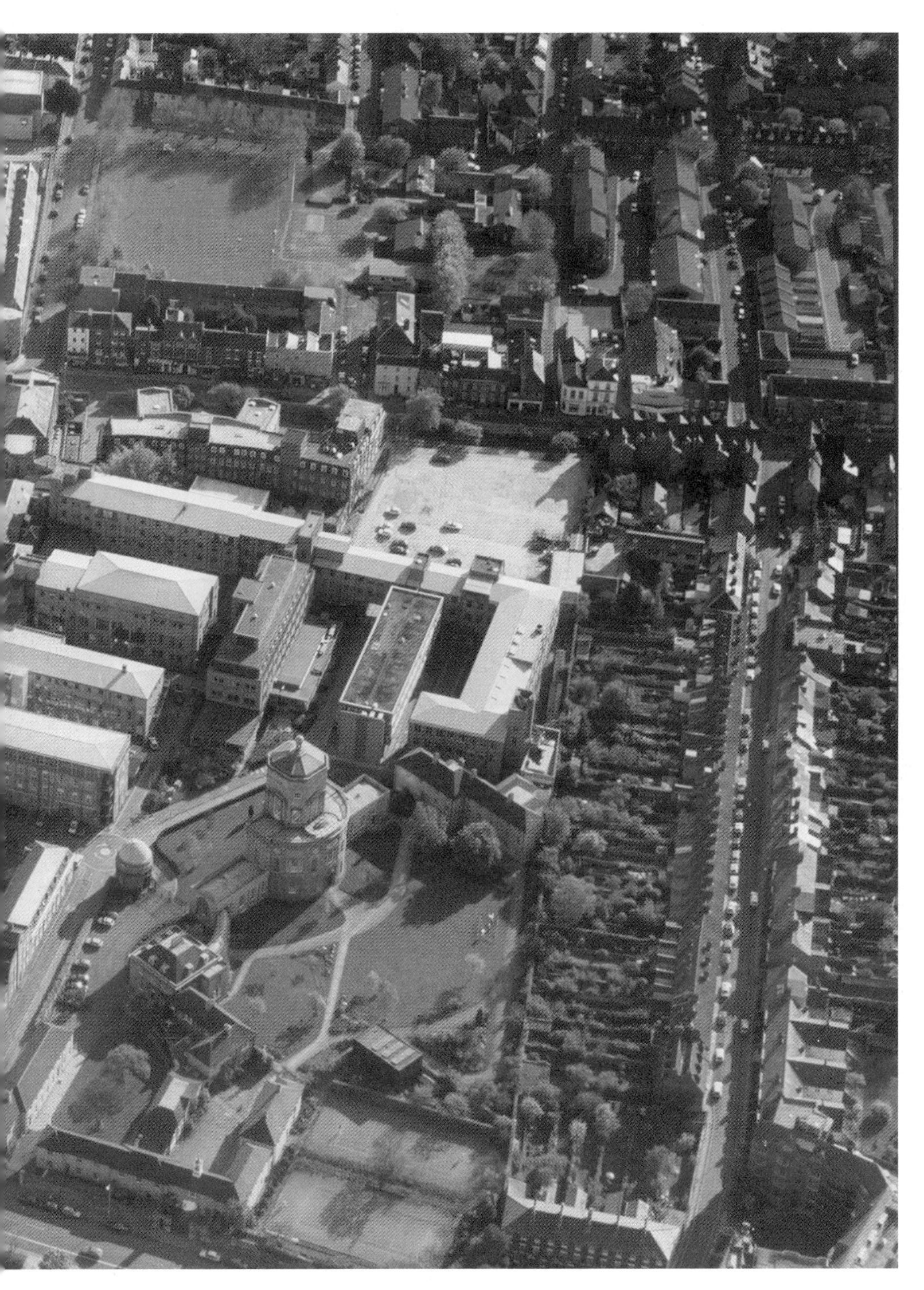

Many of the following pictures are from the *Oxford Mail and Times* and give us a glimpse of life at the RI in the past fifty years. Some are linked with items from Oxfordshire Health Archives to remind us that while some things change beyond recognition, others – like waiting to see a doctor – remained very much the same.

14 Pair Sheets Officers — Feb. ye 20. 1778 — 14 Pair
396 d° — Patients — 287
12 — Servants — 12
72 Pillow Coves — 55
6 Huckaback Round Towells — 6
71 Table Cloaths Patients & Servants — 62
54 Round Towells — 35
21 Plaine — 21
48 Shirts & Shifts & 2 Bathing D° — 48 & 2
2 Surplices — 2
2 Bed Gowns & Flannell Waiscoats & Gown — D°
2 Doz: Table Cloth 12 Napkin – Parlour — D°

Eliz: Whately
Sarah Parker

RADCLIFFE INFIRMARY
AND
COUNTY HOSPITAL,
OXFORD.

JUNE, 1909.

In presenting the second Report of the Ladies' Linen League, Mrs. Skene wishes again to thank the Vice-Presidents and their Associates for their cordial and ready help.

Mrs. Skene wishes to draw attention to the Banbury district not being properly represented. Sixty-seven In-patients were sent to the Hospital from Banbury alone, besides many Out-patients, and numerous In-patients and Out-patients from all the villages close round Banbury. Mrs. Skene hopes to receive the names of some Ladies as Vice-Presidents from this big district.

It is absolutely necessary in a large Hospital to keep the supply of linen up yearly. There are seven Wards with an average of twenty-four beds in each. An average of 10,000 articles are in the wash each week; this gives an idea of what is required. The Matron has kindly sent Mrs. Skene the following facts:

During the year 1908 there were 2,178 patients in the Hospital—the highest number on any one day being 150; and although the stock of sheets, &c., is good, we have so many cases (some only in for a day or two) that the sheets are practically on the beds, or being washed.

It was mentioned at the Annual Meeting that one lady would not subscribe because sheets were wanted again this year. Perhaps it might be pointed out that although the League provided 140 sheets, which was a very great help, still that does not mean even one sheet to a bed.

Linen and Laundry

Above: In January 1778 the governors asked for an inventory of the linen. This list, signed by Elizabeth Whately and Sarah Parker, the first two matrons, was the result. Elizabeth Whately lost her job at this time over an incident when a dead baby girl was found in the box under the wooden bed of a patient who had been admitted with a 'dropsical disorder' and gave birth to a stillborn child. Admitting pregnant women was against the rules. The fact that both matrons have signed the list suggests it may have been a 'handover' list between the two.

Left: The Ladies' Linen League was formed in 1908 to provide sheets and other items. This report from 1909 records that an average of 10,000 items were in the wash each week. During the year there were 2,178 patients and although the stock of sheets was good there were so many cases that the sheets were, 'practically on the beds or being washed'.

All linen needing mending went to the linen room. If it could not be mended it was made into sheets for the children's ward, cloths, dusters, or engine rags. The better parts were used for skin cases, for which tar ointment or gentian violet were standard treatments, leaving sheets indelibly stained.

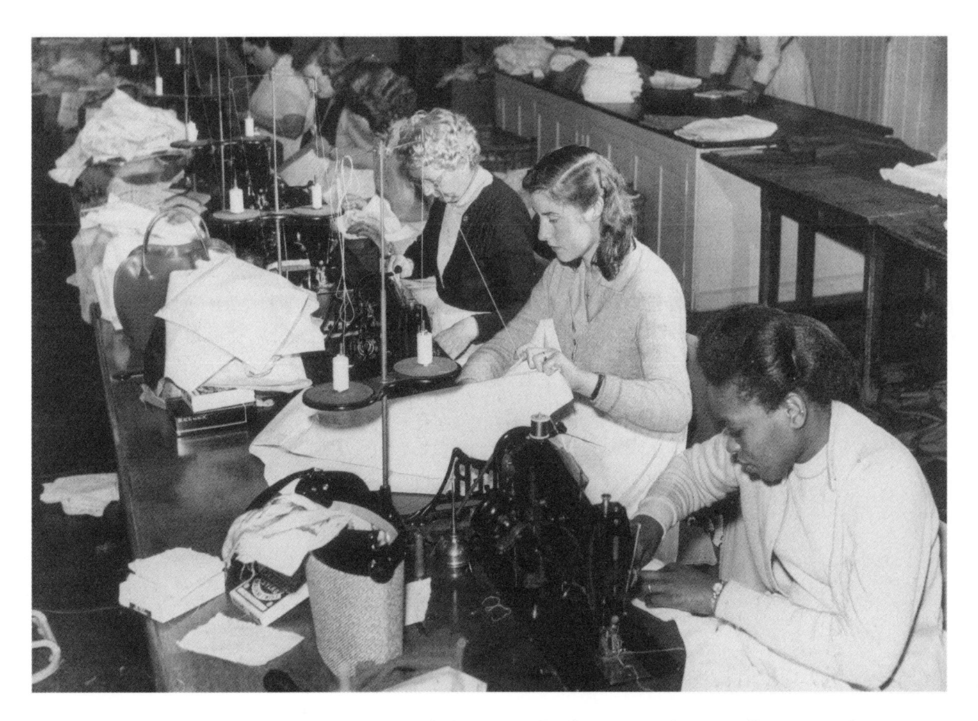

Above and below: Fifty years on, in 1959, and the same thrifty approach was still in use. Like many hospitals the Infirmary had its own laundry and a team of ladies in the sewing room. In the immediate post-war period caps and collars were still starched and ironed and white coats were so stiff they were difficult to squeeze into. (*Oxford Mail and Times*)

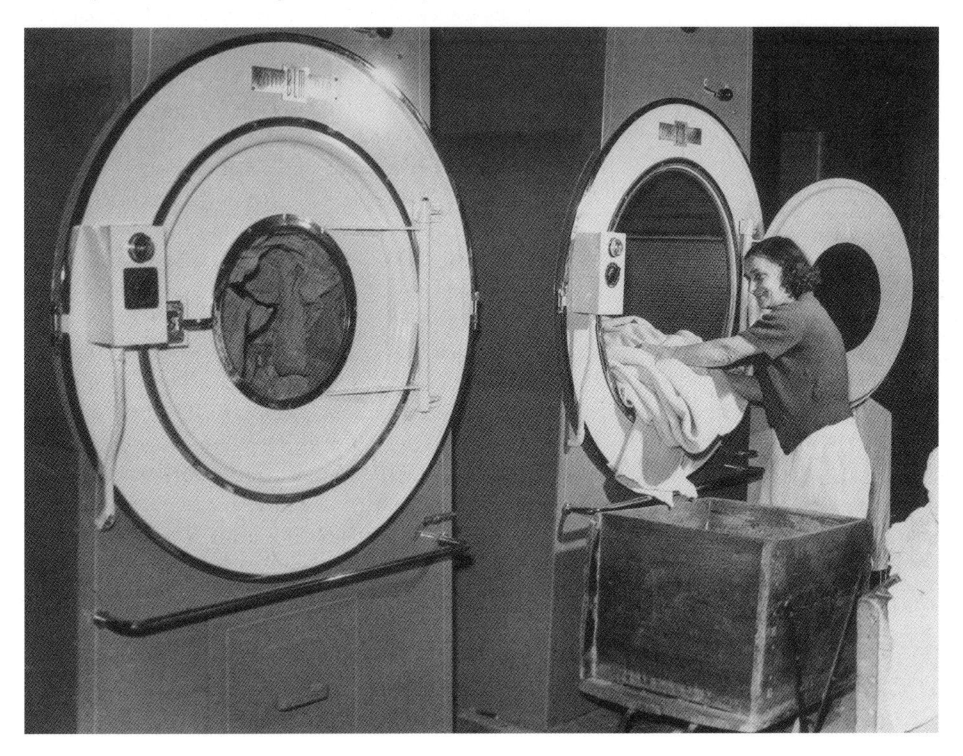

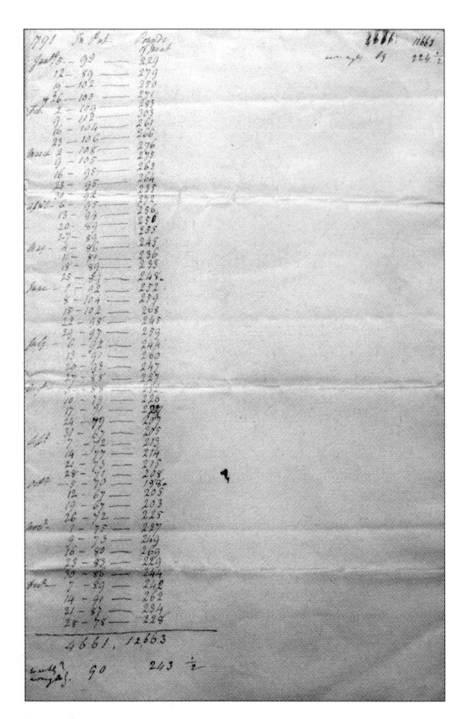

Food

Left: This list, diligently recorded in 1791, shows the weekly purchase of meat for the patients. During that year the Infirmary bought 12,663 pounds of meat at a cost of £4,661.

Below: Approved diets for early nineteenth-century patients, according to their condition. Water gruel was part of the diet for everyone. Meals were eaten from wooden or pewter vessels with earthenware mugs for the daily ration of beer, which was brewed on the premises until 1853.

A TABLE OF DIET.

Common or House Diet.

SUNDAY and THURSDAY.

Breakfast,—Water-gruel, or Milk-pottage, a pint.
Dinner,—Veal or Mutton boiled, five ounces, and a pint of Broth.
Supper,—SUNDAY, Cheese two ounces, or Butter one ounce. THURSDAY, Water-gruel, Milk-pottage, or Broth, a pint.

MONDAY and FRIDAY.

Breakfast,—Milk-pottage, Water-gruel, or Broth, a pint.
Dinner,—Rice-milk, a pint.
Supper,—Cheese two ounces, or Butter one ounce.

TUESDAY and SATURDAY.

Breakfast,—Water-gruel, or Milk-pottage, a pint.
Dinner,—Mutton or Beef boiled, five ounces, and a pint of Broth.
Supper,—Water-gruel, Milk-pottage, or Broth, a pint.

WEDNESDAY.

Breakfast,—Milk-pottage, or Water-gruel, a pint.
Dinner,—Bread-pudding baked, ten ounces.
Supper,—Cheese two ounces, or Butter one ounce.

Beer, SUNDAY, MONDAY, WEDNESDAY, and FRIDAY, three half pints a day. TUESDAY, THURSDAY, and SATURDAY, a pint a day.

Full Diet.

SUNDAY and THURSDAY.

Breakfast,—Water-gruel, or Milk-pottage, a pint.
Dinner,—Veal or Mutton boiled, eight ounces.
Supper,—SUNDAY, Cheese two ounces, or Butter one ounce. THURSDAY, Water-gruel, Milk-pottage, or Broth, a pint.

MONDAY and FRIDAY.

Breakfast,—Milk-pottage, Water-gruel, or Broth, a pint.
Dinner,—Rice-milk, a pint.
Supper,—Cheese two ounces, or Butter one ounce.

TUESDAY and SATURDAY.

Breakfast,—Water-gruel, or Milk-pottage, a pint.
Dinner,—Mutton or Beef boiled, eight ounces.
Supper,—Water-gruel, Milk-pottage, or Broth, a pint.

WEDNESDAY.

Breakfast,—Milk-pottage, or Water-gruel, a pint.
Dinner,—Bread-pudding baked, 12 ounces.
Supper,—Cheese two ounces, or Butter one ounce.

Beer, SUNDAY, MONDAY, WEDNESDAY, and FRIDAY, a quart a day. TUESDAY, THURSDAY, and SATURDAY, three half pints a day.

Low Diet.

SUNDAY and THURSDAY.

Breakfast,—Water-gruel, or Milk-pottage, a pint.
Dinner,—Veal or Mutton boiled, two ounces, and a pint of Broth.
Supper,—SUNDAY, Cheese two ounces, or Butter one ounce. THURSDAY, Water-gruel, Milk-pottage, or Broth, a pint.

MONDAY and FRIDAY.

Breakfast,—Milk-pottage, or Water-gruel, a pint.
Dinner,—Rice-milk, a pint.
Supper,—Cheese two ounces, or Butter one ounce.

TUESDAY and SATURDAY.

Breakfast,—Water-gruel, or Milk-pottage, a pint.
Dinner,—Mutton or Beef boiled, two ounces, and a pint of Broth.
Supper,—Water-gruel, Milk-pottage, or Broth, a pint.

WEDNESDAY.

Breakfast,—Milk-pottage, or Water-gruel, a pint.
Dinner,—Bread-pudding baked, eight ounces.
Supper,—Cheese two ounces, or Butter one ounce.

Beer, SUNDAY, MONDAY, WEDNESDAY, and FRIDAY, three half pints a day. TUESDAY, THURSDAY, and SATURDAY, a pint a day.

Fever Diet.

Barley-water, Water-gruel, Panado, thin Broth, Milk-pottage, Sagoe, Rice-gruel, Balm or Sage Tea, when ordered.

Milk Diet.

SUNDAY, TUESDAY, THURSDAY, and SATURDAY.

Breakfast,—Milk-pottage, or Water-gruel, a pint.
Dinner,—Rice-milk, a pint.
Supper,—Milk-pottage, or Water-gruel, a pint.

MONDAY.

Breakfast,—Milk-pottage, or Water-gruel, a pint.
Dinner,—Bread-pudding 8 ounces.
Supper,—Water-gruel, or Milk-pottage, a pint.

WEDNESDAY and FRIDAY.

Breakfast,—Water-gruel, or Milk-pottage, a pint.
Dinner,—Bread-pudding 8 ounces.
Supper,—Butter one ounce.

Drink, three pints in a day, one part Milk and two Water.

Dry Diet.

SUNDAY and THURSDAY.

Breakfast,—Cheese two ounces, or Butter one ounce.
Dinner,—Veal or Mutton roasted, six ounces.
Supper,—Cheese two ounces, or Butter one ounce.

MONDAY, WEDNESDAY, and FRIDAY.

Breakfast,—Cheese two ounces, or Butter one ounce.
Dinner,—Rice-pudding well baked, eight ounces.
Supper,—Cheese two ounces, or Butter one ounce.

TUESDAY and SATURDAY.

Breakfast,—Cheese two ounces, or Butter one ounce.
Dinner,—Mutton roasted, six ounces.
Supper,—Cheese two ounces, or Butter one ounce.

Beer, three half pints a day.—If Sea-biscuits can conveniently be had, the Patients may be allowed them sufficient, without waste.

RULES to be observed in the TABLES of DIET.

IN the Common or House Diet, it is to be understood, that half a pound of raw Meat is allowed to every Patient, which, when dressed, will produce Broth of a sufficient strength; and the Meat remaining being divided will amount to about five ounces for every Patient, exclusive of bones.

Three pounds of Meat are to be added to every gallon of Broth for Patients on the Low Diet.

All Patients are allowed Bread sufficient, without waste.

All Patients, at their first admission into the House, are to be put upon the Common House Diet, except the contrary is ordered by the Physician or Surgeon attending them.

Grosvenor and Hall, Printers, Oxford.

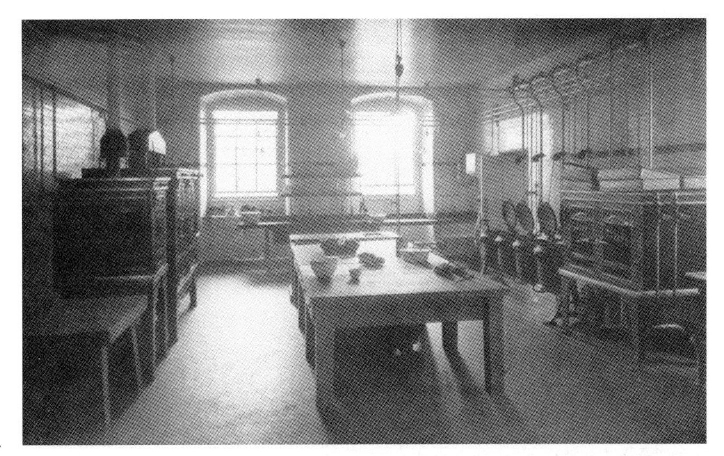
The new kitchen in 1906.

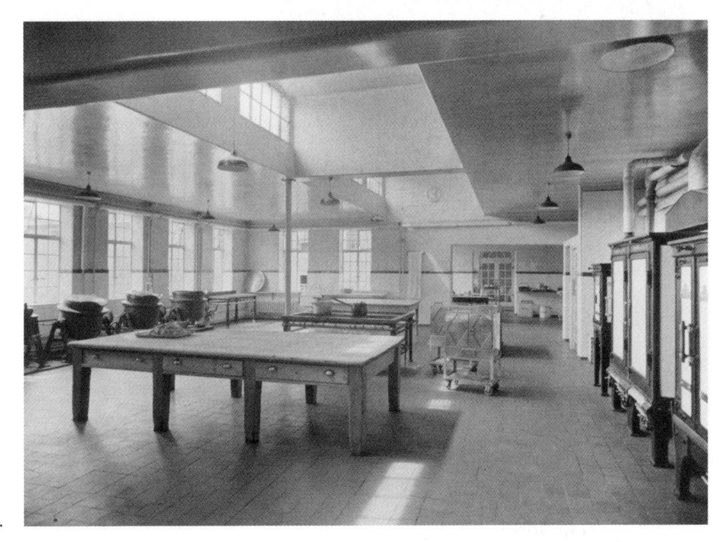
The kitchen, *c.* 1935.

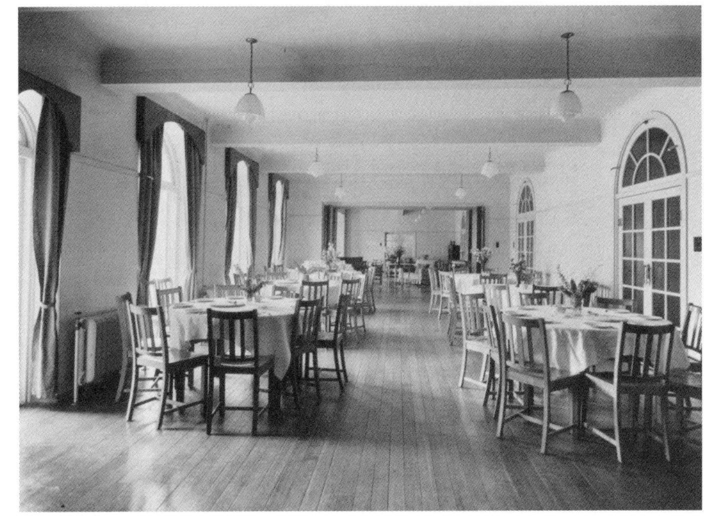
The nurses' dining room, *c.* 1935.

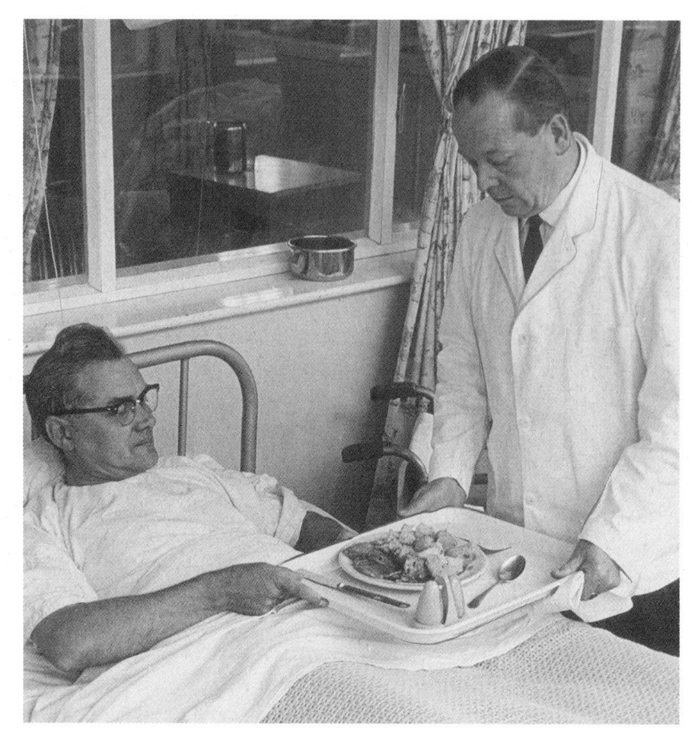

Left: An experiment was introduced in Cronshaw ward in 1964 when catering staff took over serving food to patients. Catering manager Mr F.H. Bavin said it was one of the most important factors in patient–hospital relationships. (*Oxford Mail and Times*)

Below: A new restaurant opened in 1966, replacing five separate dining rooms for medical, nursing and lay staff. It was now national policy to have a single restaurant for all grades. The new kitchen had stainless steel equipment and lunch was 2*s* 7*d*. (*Oxford Mail and Times*)

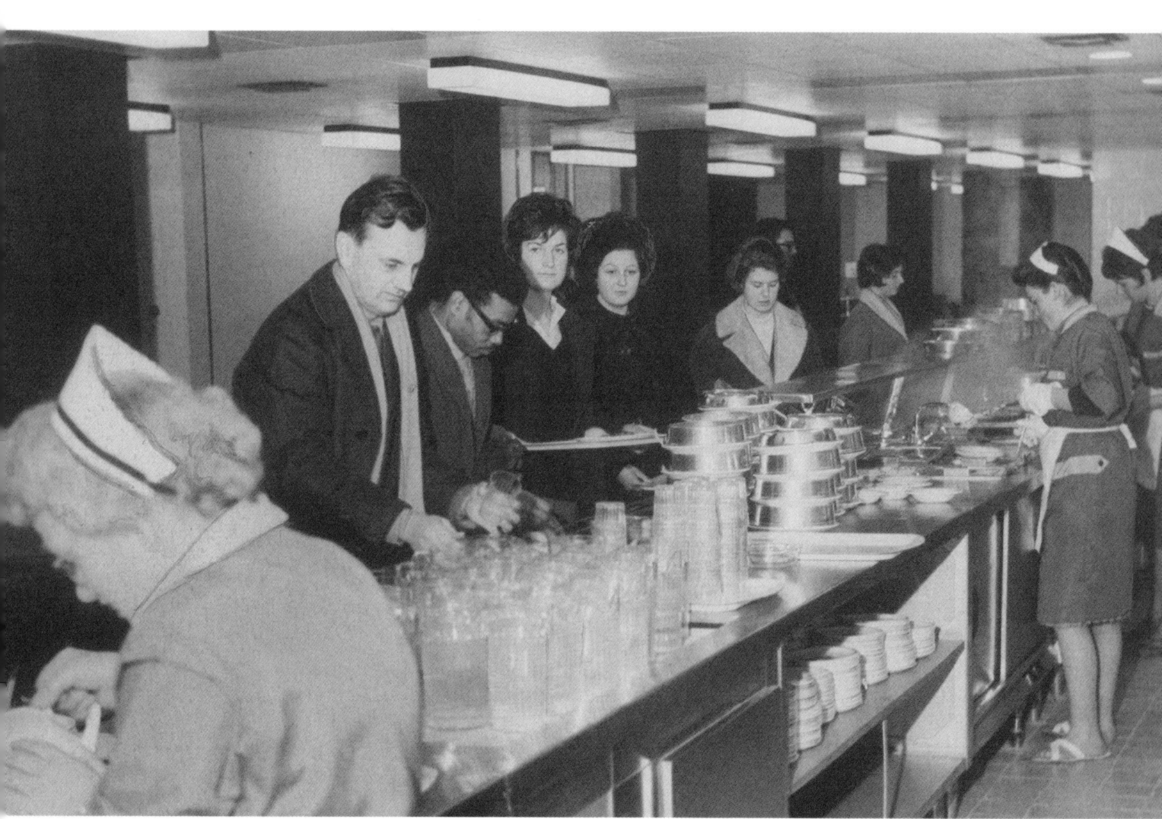

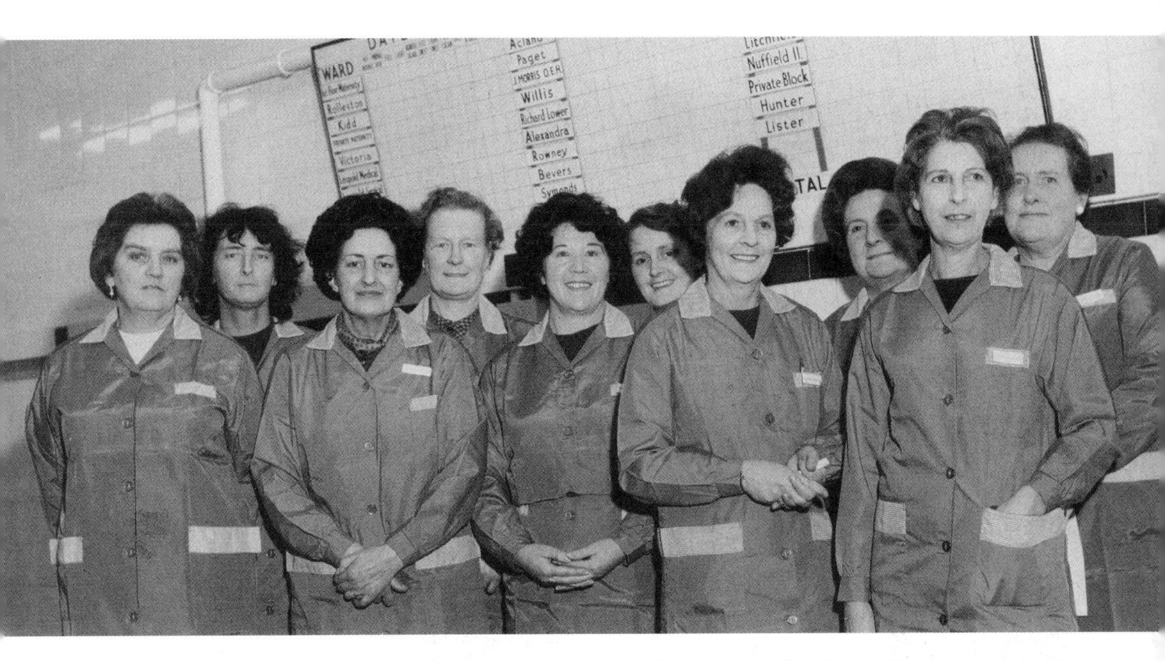

Ward hostesses line up for the camera in 1967 when the RI became the first hospital in Europe to use entirely frozen food catering. Patients were said to be impressed with tasty roast beef, Yorkshire pudding and roast potatoes on the first day. (*Oxford Mail and Times*)

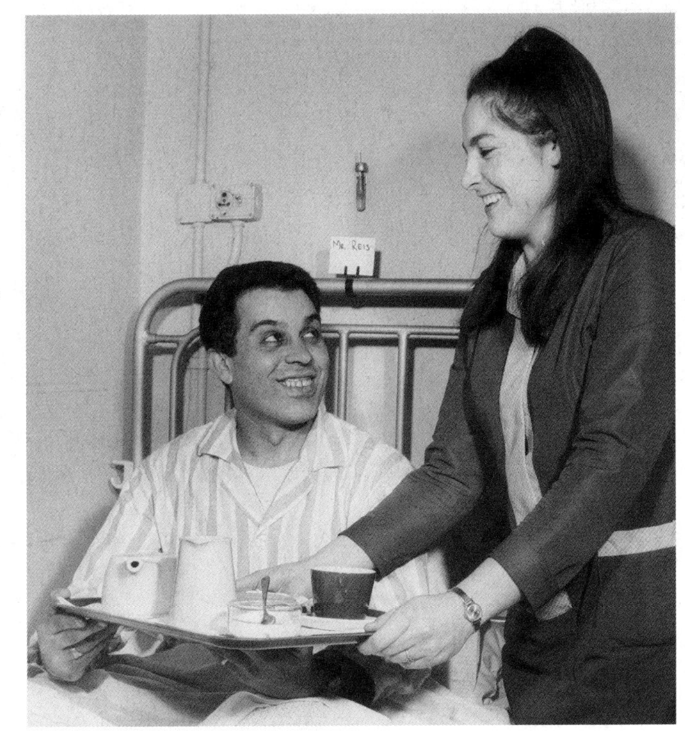

In the late 1960s the Radcliffe Infirmary adopted the new idea of employing housekeepers and ward assistants who would relieve nurses of duties such as bedmaking, serving food, answering the phone and looking after visitors so that the nurses could concentrate on more skilled work.

They were first introduced on Lichfield ward in 1968 and were so successful the governors allocated an extra £9,000 in 1969 to extend the scheme. Alexandra, Symonds, Rowney and Bevers wards each had four ward assistants in blue and white dress uniforms, a housekeeper and assistant housekeeper. (*Oxford Mail and Times*)

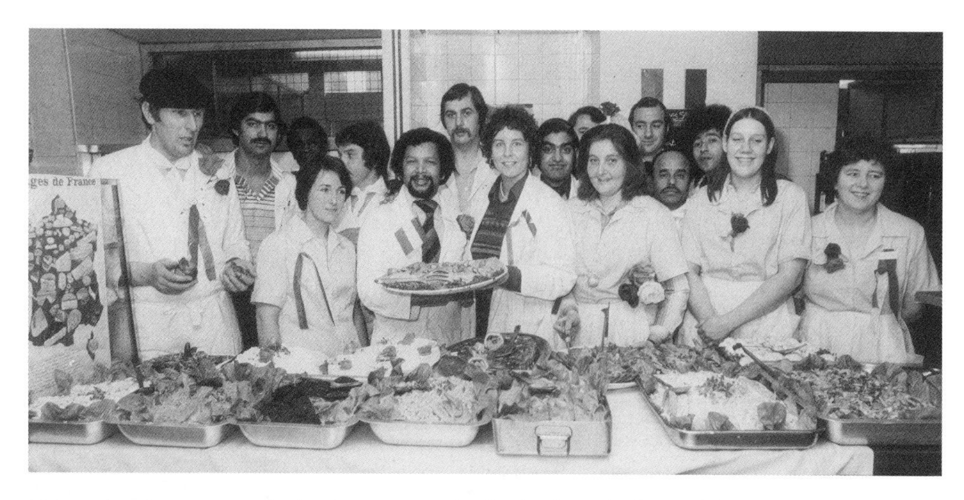

Theme days became popular in the restaurant in the 1970s as the hospital began to employ a more cosmopolitan staff. This was a French theme day set up by catering manager Jane Reast (centre). (*Oxford Mail and Times*)

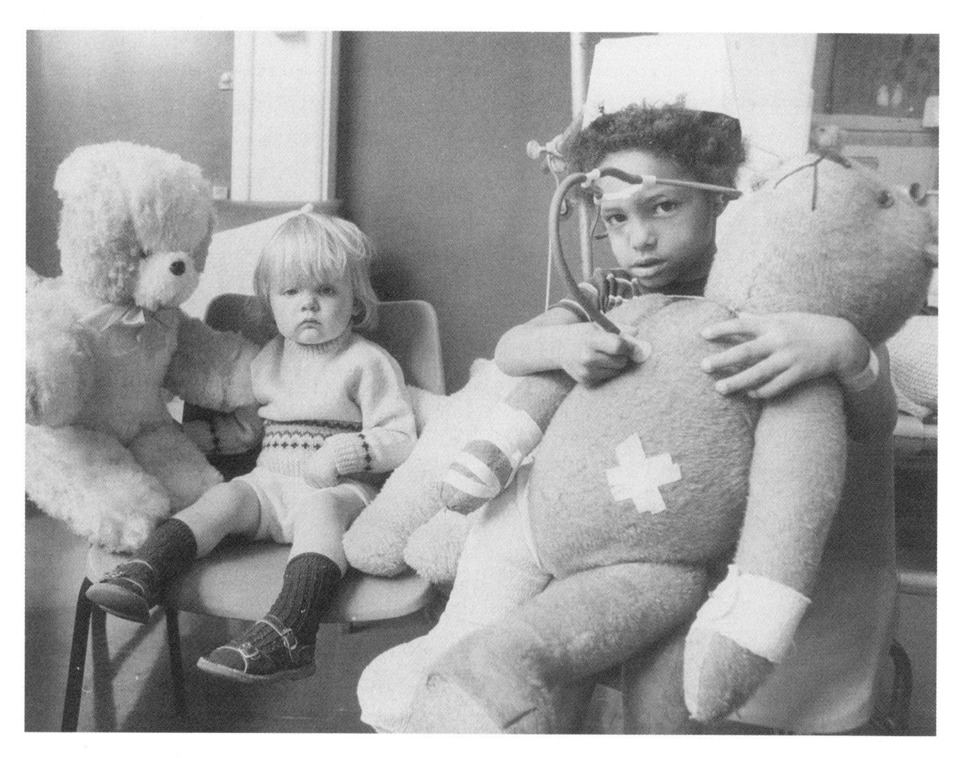

Teddy goes to hospital – long before hospital play specialists began using their skills to calm children's fears, nurses were using the same idea in a less systematic way. In 1972 the *Oxford Times* published a letter from Lady Ogilvie, chairman of the League of Friends, appealing for a large teddy bear which children could bandage, stitch and even inject, to help overcome their anxieties. The result was Edward Bear, aged fifty, seen here with Alex (twenty-two months) and Mark (five). The bear became a fixture on Leopold ward, replacing an older one which had fallen to bits. (*Oxford Mail and Times*)

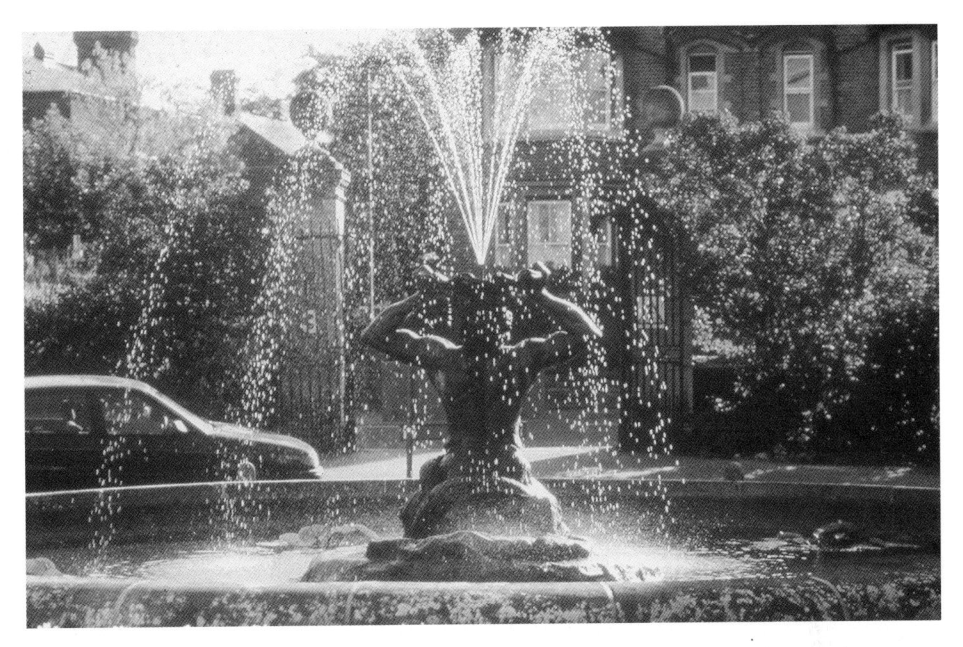

The Triton fountain in the front courtyard has been a popular meeting place, backdrop for photographs and refuge for nearly 150 years since it was installed in 1857. Triton was the son of Neptune in Greek mythology, and had the body of a man and the tail of a fish. The figure is the work of John Bell, a distinguished sculptor, and was made in terracotta by J.M. Blashfield of Praed Street, Paddington.

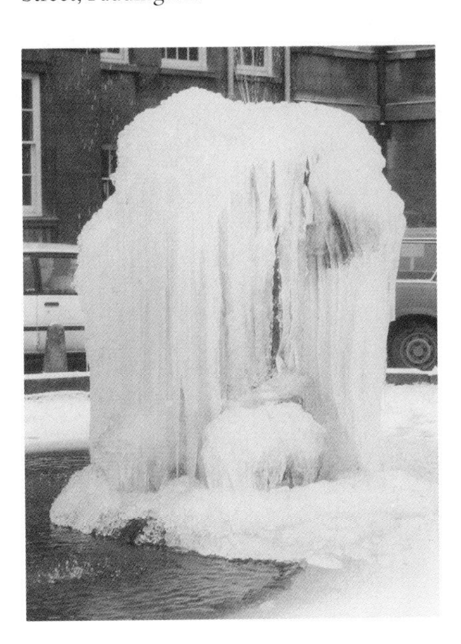

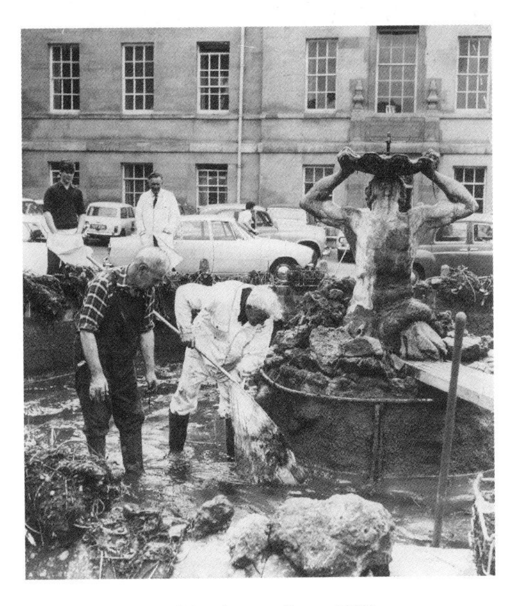

Above left: In severe weather it is often festooned with ice, as in this picture from 1985.

Above right: Work to remove decades of accumulated mud and repair a leak in May 1971. More than 100 goldfish were removed and returned afterwards. Arthur Merritt (in white coat), a retired hospital porter whose hobby was fish, returned to look after the evacuation. (*Oxford Mail and Times*)

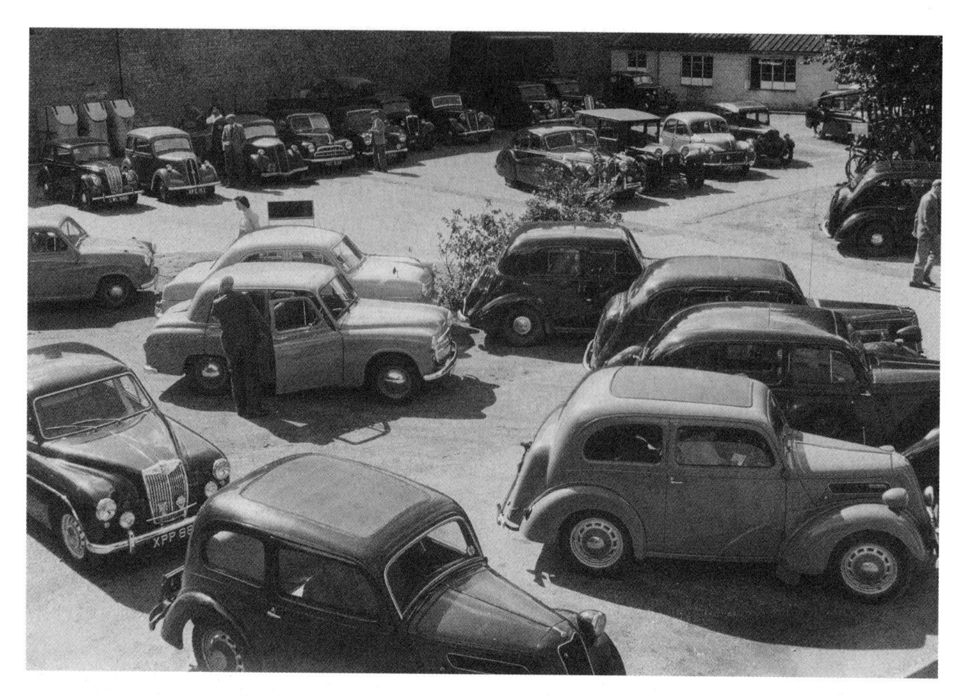

Above: Some things never change. The Radcliffe Infirmary has always had limited space for parking, although in 1956 when this picture was taken fewer members of staff would have had cars. Even so, the car park looks full enough. (*Oxford Mail and Times*)

Below: Parking became more and more difficult to manage as car ownership increased. This traffic census in 1963 aimed to check the extent of 'unofficial' parking. (*Oxford Mail and Times*)

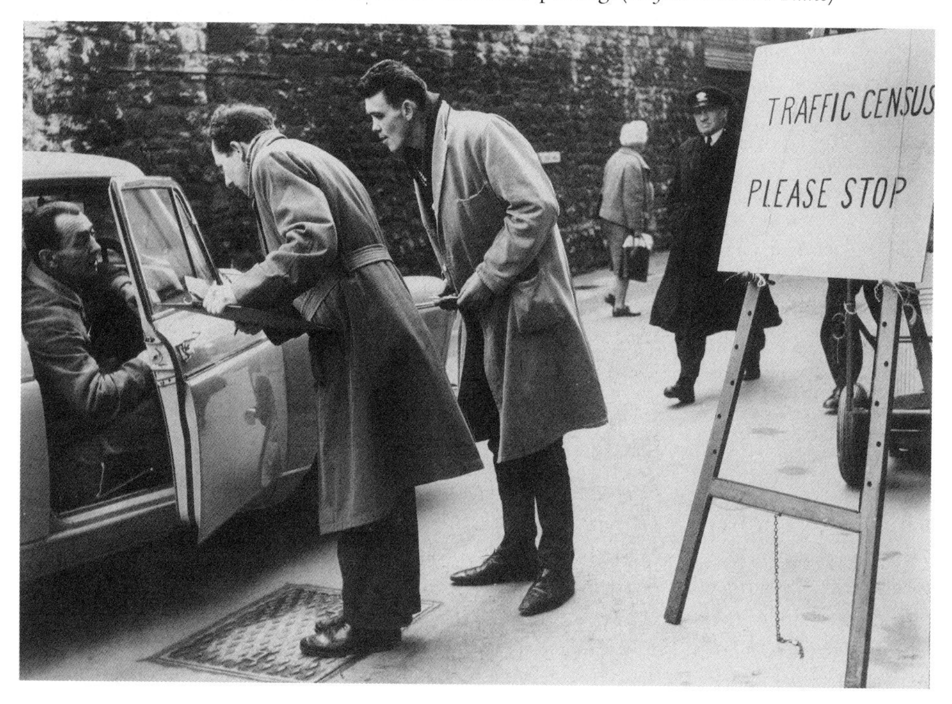

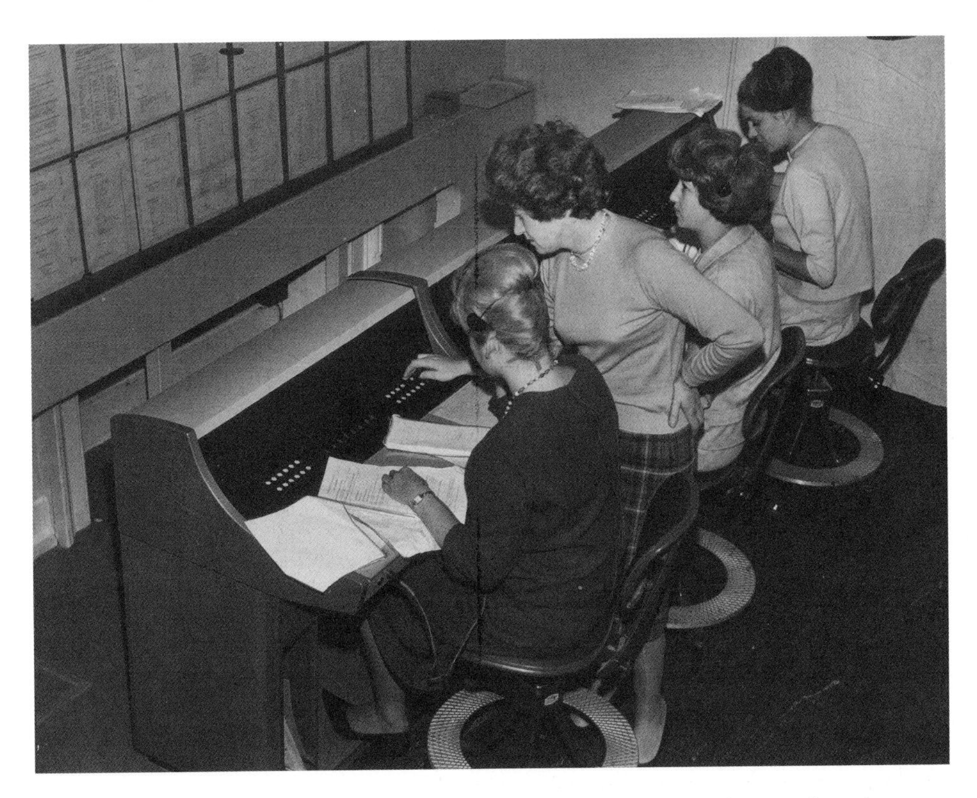

The first telephone was installed outside the accident ward in 1899 and a few years later they were in use throughout the hospital – although patients complained about the noise of the bells and they had to be muffled.

This £25,000 cordless console was the latest thing in phone technology when it was introduced in 1963. The hospital now had 650 phones compared with 350 and internal calls could be dialled direct instead of through the switchboard. (*Oxford Mail and Times*)

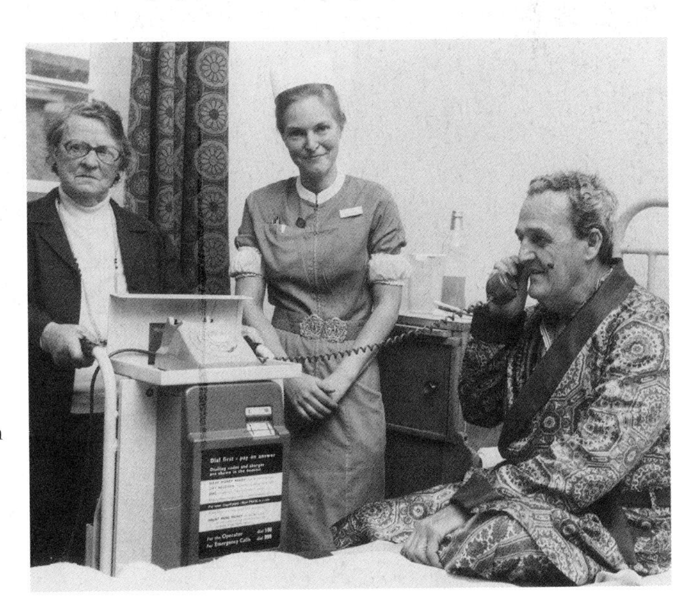

'Mobile' phones began to make an appearance in the hospital in the 1970s – Post Office pay phones on a trolley that could be wheeled to the bedside. This one, being used by patient Mr Gordon Smith on Bevers ward, was bought by the Post Office Engineering Union for £80 in memory of a former branch chairman. The nurse is Sister Margaret Uttley. (*Oxford Mail and Times*)

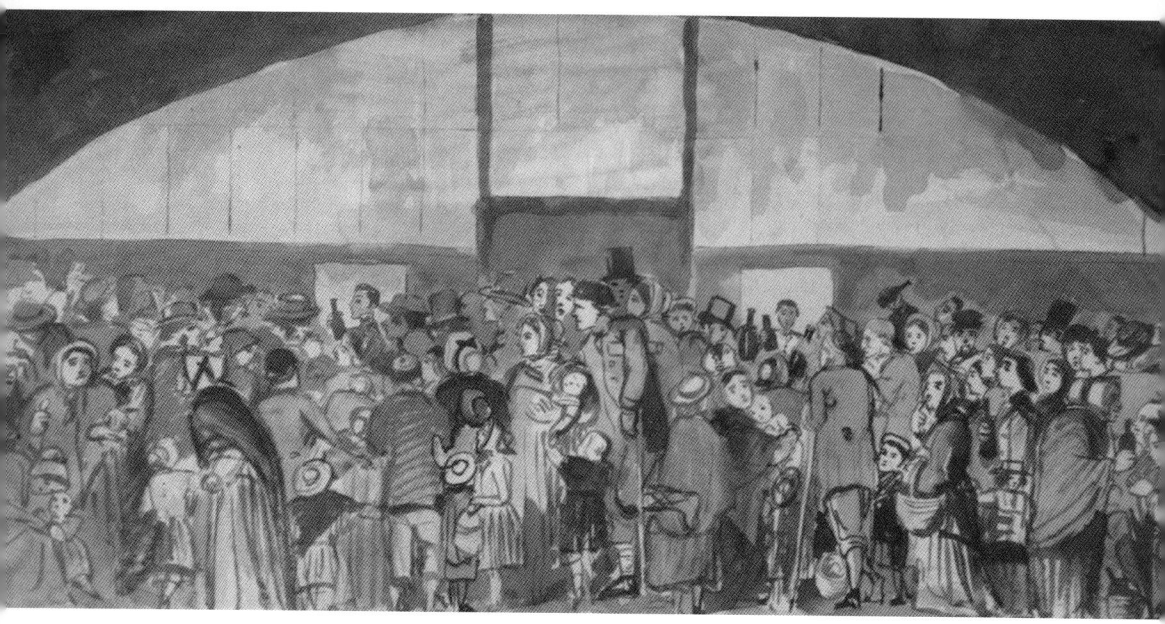

Waiting

A watercolour of the waiting hall, *c.*1860. Acland was so concerned by the numbers of people that he arranged for Miss Mary Severn (Mrs Charles Newton) to make a scale drawing of the crowd. The artist, whose father was a friend of the poet Keats, said there were twenty-five more people than the picture actually shows.

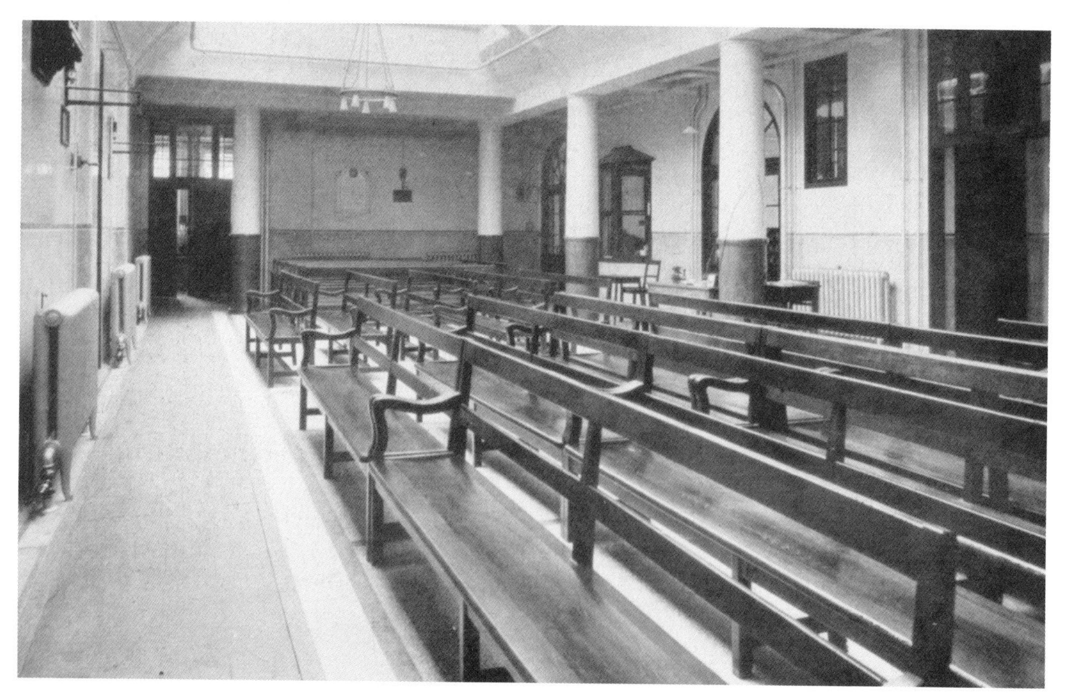

The main outpatients waiting hall, *c.* 1909.

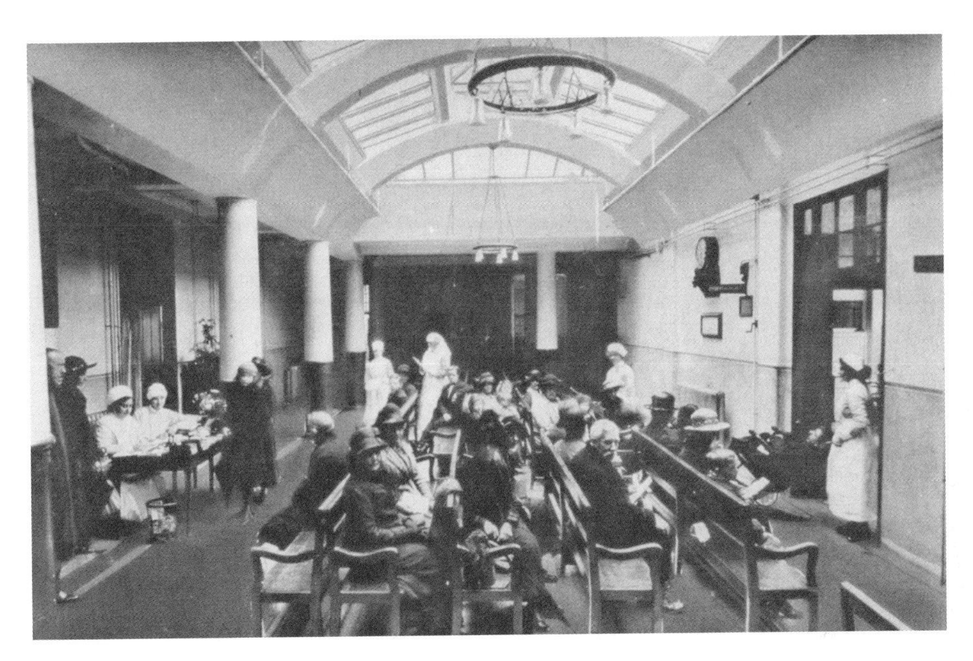

The outpatients waiting hall, *c.* 1920…

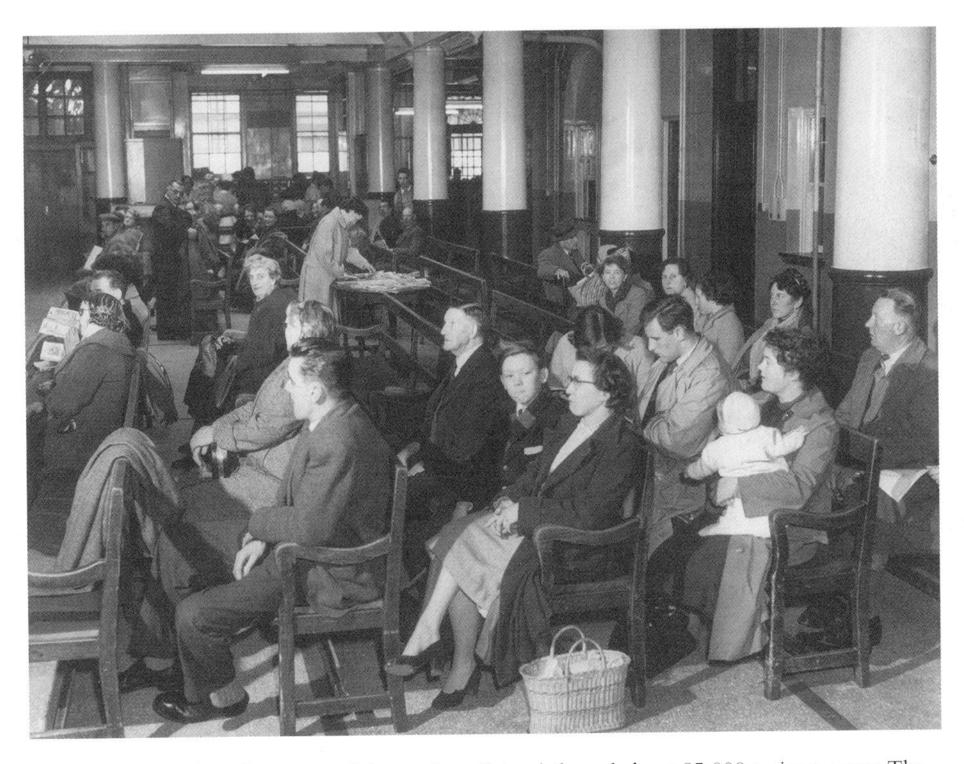

… and in 1959 when there were eight or nine clinics daily and about 85,000 patients a year. The benches on which the patients sit quietly waiting were the same as those in use fifty years earlier. They later made their way to other parts of the hospital where they provided a resting place for weary visitors. (*Oxford Mail and Times*)

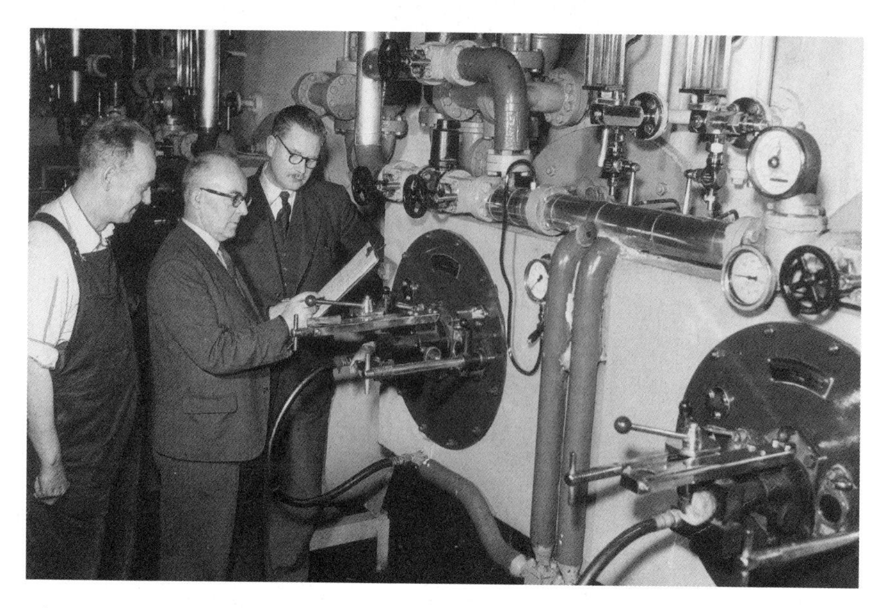

The *Oxford Times* interviewed the Infirmary's building supervisor, Mr R.A. Johnson, and superintendent engineer, Mr G.F.P. Henagulph in 1959 about their work to keep the hospital running smoothly amid constant change. Mr Johnson told the paper that in the past fifteen years he had seen the hospital grow by nearly a third. At the time nearly 400 people lived in and there were twenty-six wards with up to 600 patients.

The engineers were responsible for all the steam, hot water, electricity, sterilising, piped oxygen, laundry and the maintenance of all hospital services. In this picture Mr Henagulph (centre) and Mr Johnson (right) are inspecting the boiler house that was converted from coal to oil burning in 1955. (*Oxford Mail and Times*)

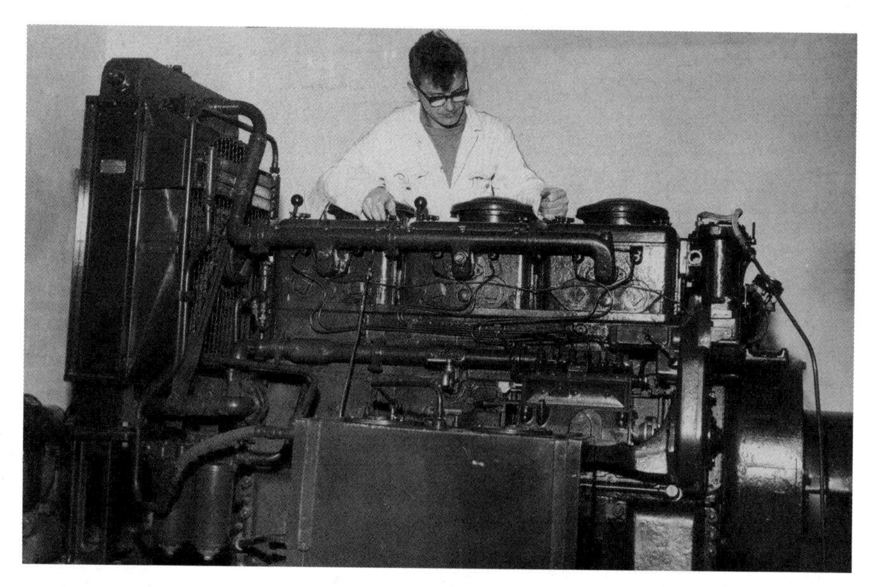

Gas and electricity supplies were sometimes uncertain in the cold winters of the early 1960s. But this standby generator being tended by maintenance electrician Denis Farndell was on hand to keep services going if the mains supply failed. (*Oxford Mail and Times*)

eight

Advances and Discoveries

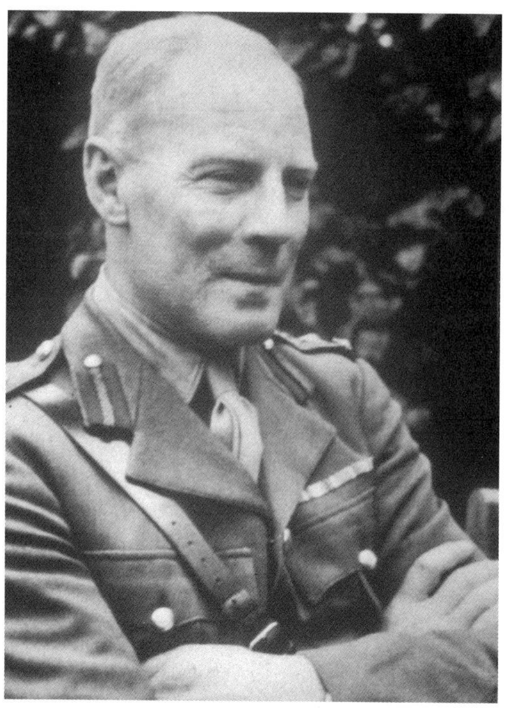

Sir Hugh Cairns 1896-1952
He was an Australian-born brain surgeon who had been called to the bedside of Lawrence of Arabia after his fatal motorcycle accident in 1935. Appointed the first Nuffield Professor of Surgery at Oxford in 1937, his wartime research on the causes of death among motorcyclists showed the lifesaving value of crash helmets, but it was thirty-two years after his first paper that they became compulsory. As well as being one of the leading neurosurgeons of his day, he played an important part in the success of the first accident department.

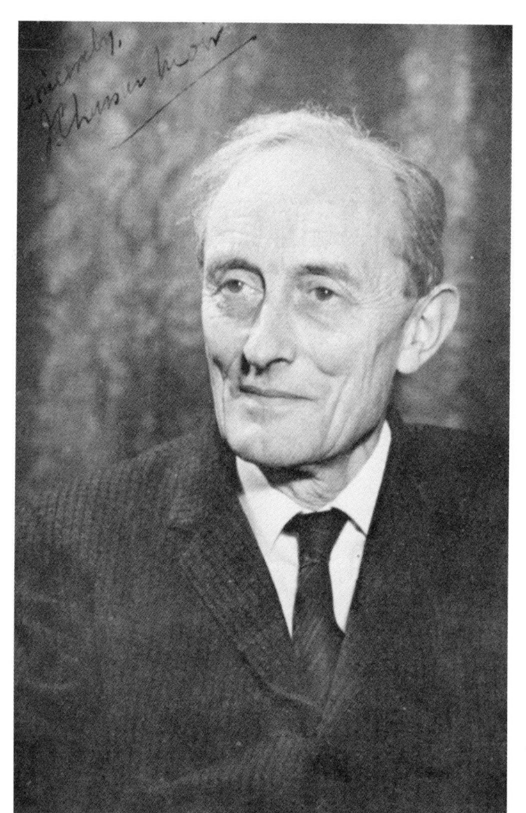

Chassar Moir 1900-1977
He was the first Nuffield Professor of Obstetrics and Gynaecology. A scholarly man with a record of outstanding medical and surgical advances behind him, he was a painstaking and meticulous surgeon, renowned for his gentleness and approachability.

With his eager colleague John (later Sir John) Stallworthy, he established an obstetric flying squad with doctors and nurses on twenty-four-hour standby to go out to mothers in crisis during childbirth instead of having them brought in near death. Over the next thirty-five years the squad went to the aid of over 2,000 mothers and saved all but one. Other hospitals quickly copied the idea.

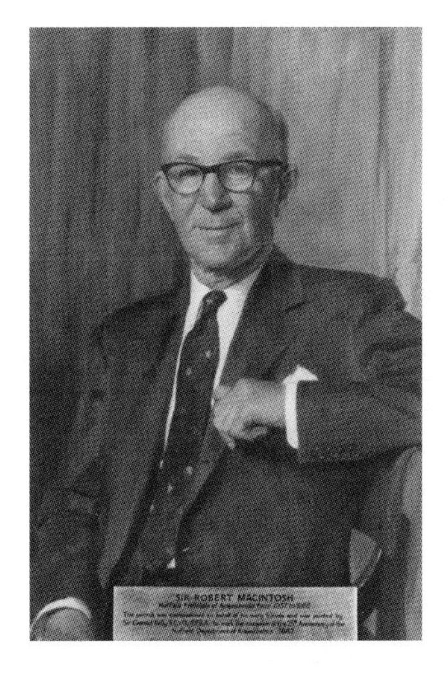

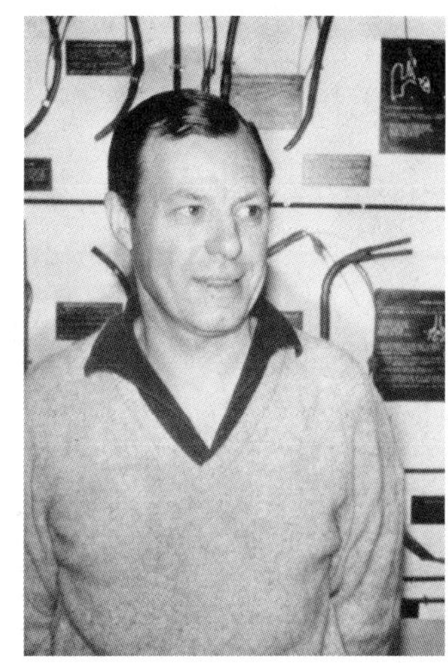

Right: Sir Robert Macintosh was appointed the first Professor of Anaesthetics in Europe when Lord Nuffield made his famous benefaction. At first the university turned down the idea because it considered anaesthetics a craft for medical artisans who liked gadgets and not worthy of scholarly attention. But Nuffield made it clear that without anaesthetics the other professorships were at risk and it was quickly accepted.

Initially working in huts and workshops, Macintosh advanced his speciality to a department of worldwide acclaim, with a prolific output of research and a series of inventions of both simple and sophisticated apparatus.

Far right: The development of anaesthetics was carried a stage further by Professor Alex Crampton Smith whose work on respiratory problems, in harness with neurologist John Spalding, saved many lives of patients with polio or tetanus, through the use of the intermittent positive pressure pump.

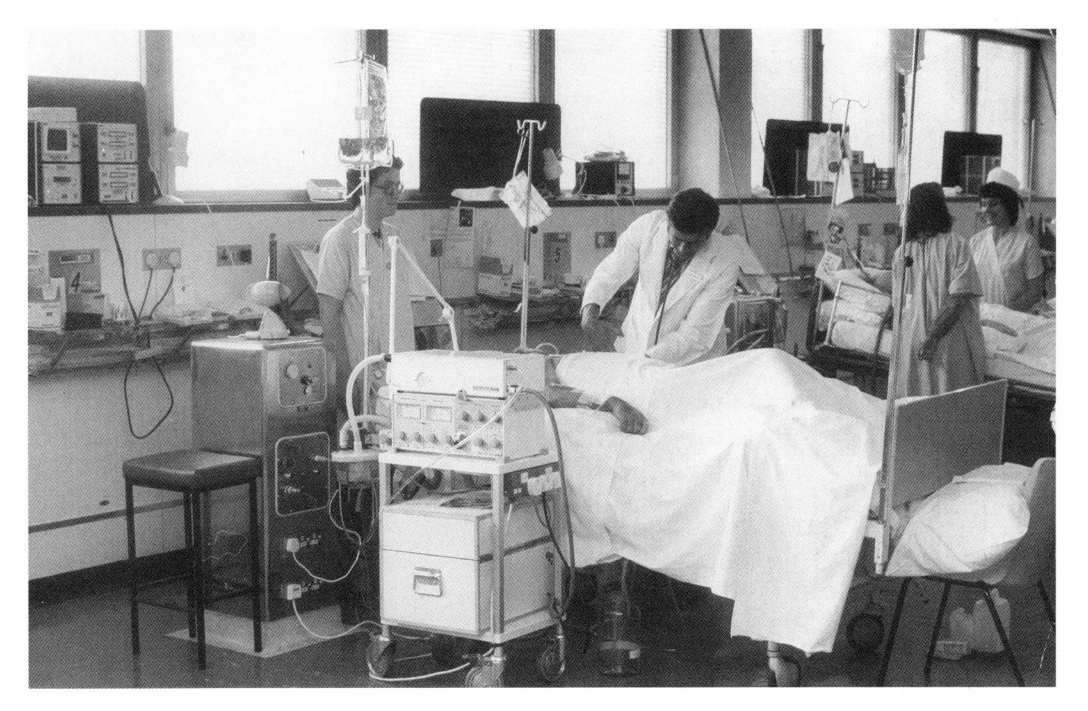

An intensive care unit opened in the early 1970s and by the end of the decade the technology had moved on and consultant anaesthetist Dr Anthony Fisher (pictured) was backing a fund-raising appeal for equipment such as ventilators to keep Oxford at the forefront of modern medicine. About 500 patients a year were being cared for in the unit at that time, and 85 per cent of them survived. (*Oxford Mail and Times*)

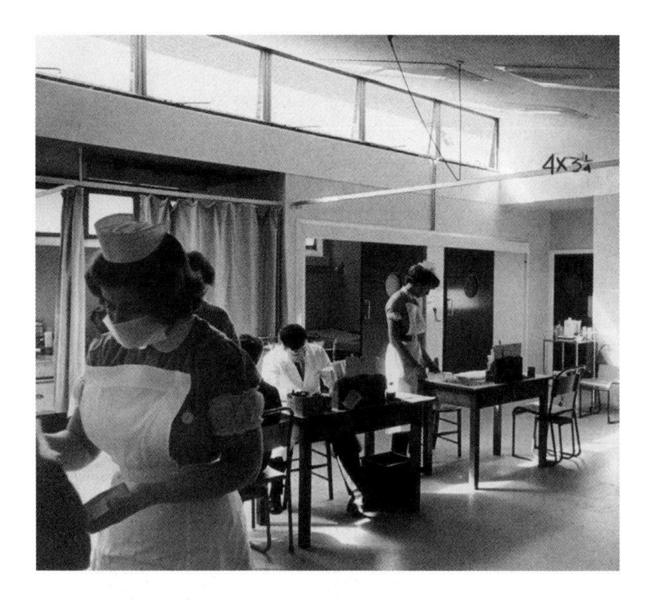

The first accident service in Britain opened at the Infirmary in 1941, initially in a single room in casualty with a small outpatient theatre, sixty surgical beds and a tiny office. It was set up by the Canadian surgeon Jim Scott and became an immediate success. Improvements in 1958 were followed by modernisation in 1964. It closed in July 1979 when the service moved to the John Radcliffe. The picture shows the new treatment room in 1964. (*Oxford Mail and Times*)

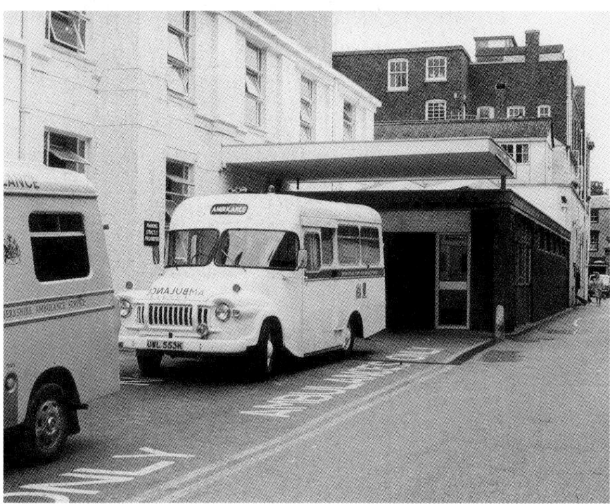

Left: The casualty department entrance, *c.* 1973.

Below left: The department, *c.*1973.

Below right: Student nurse Helen Westley closes the doors on the emergency admissions area in 1979. Formerly Bagot and Drake wards, it was the only part of the hospital which had been used continuously for treating patients for over 200 years. (*Oxford Mail and Times*)

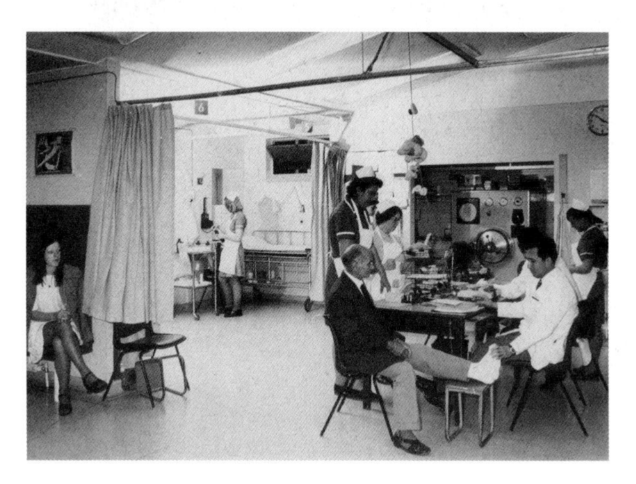

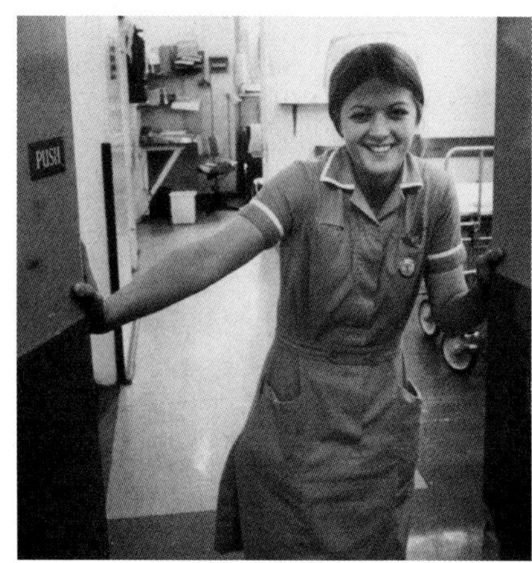

Penicillin

Among the many discoveries and innovations on which the Radcliffe Infirmary led the world, the greatest must surely have been the use of penicillin in the treatment of infections.

Years of 'brilliant and laborious work' by Howard Florey and his colleagues in the Sir William Dunn School of Pathology had succeeded in taking Sir Alexander Fleming's earlier discovery of the properties of penicillin mould to the stage where penicillin could be injected into patients.

In 1941 came the moment to test whether it would give the body the power to fight back against infection. The results were spectacular. A forty-three-year-old policeman in Briscoe ward who had been seriously ill showed a marked improvement within twenty-four hours. Although he died after treatment stopped, the team had seen enough to know that this was a major breakthrough. Muriel Flack, who nursed the patients who received those first doses, is still alive and lives in Australia.

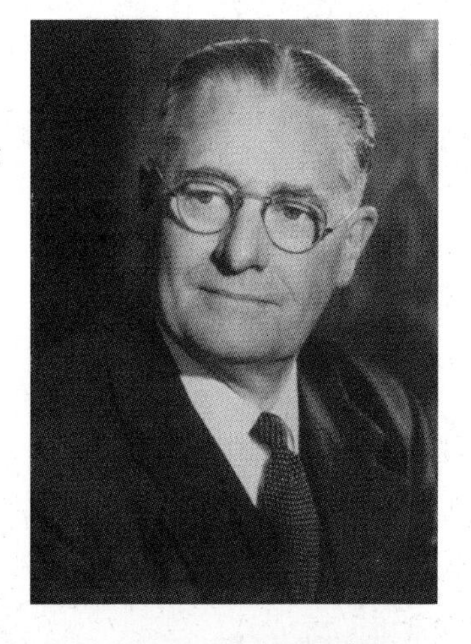

Right: Lord Florey 1898-1968
He was a key player in the hospital's most famous 'first', having qualities of great industry and determination which he drew on in the long struggle to harness the discovery.

Below: Lady Florey unveils a plaque in 1969 to commemorate the first use of penicillin for the treatment of infection at the Radcliffe Infirmary. Legend has it that the wording should have read 'systemic' (i.e. within the body's system) but an enterprising stonemason or typist managed to change it to 'systematic' (in a planned and logical pattern) on the plaque. Either seems appropriate and the plaque has remained with its original wording. (*Oxford Mail and Times*)

Penicillin made in
the Sir William Dunn School of
Pathology was first used for systematic
treatment of infection in man
in the Radcliffe Infirmary
on 12 February 1941

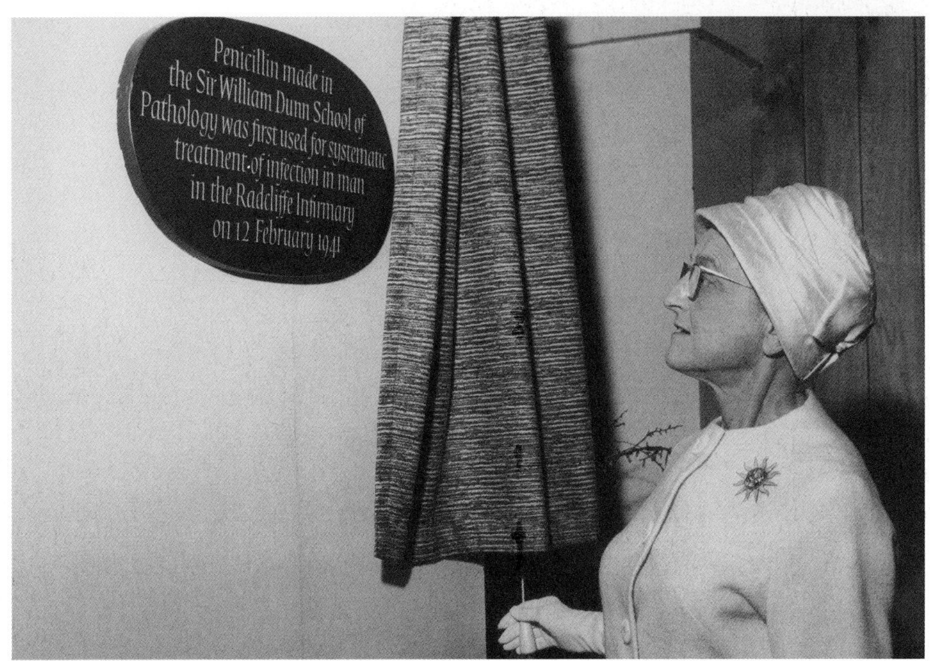

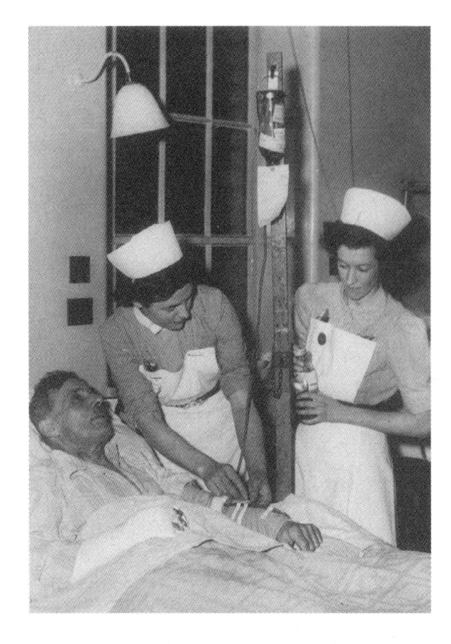

Sister Barbara Twining adjusts a drip, *c.* 1950. In 1942, when she was at the Wingfield Morris Orthopaedic Centre (now the Nuffield Orthopaedic Centre), she was sister in charge of a ward where penicillin was given to a young boy. Her detailed notes of the time record the astonishment at his rapid improvement. They are now in the Bodleian Library.

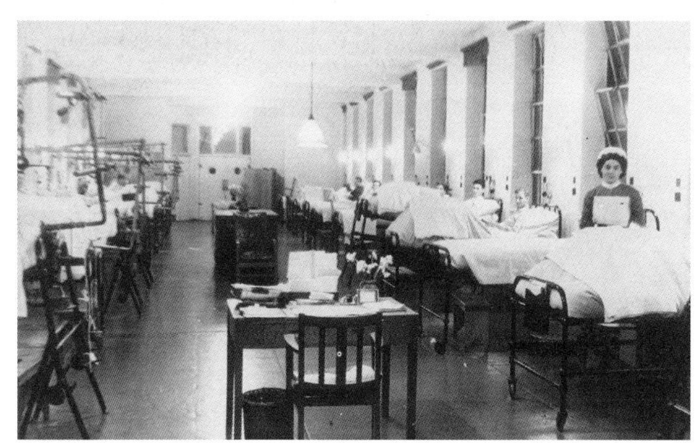

Cronshaw ward, *c.* 1950. Barbara Twining was a member of the tea family and sister on Cronshaw ward almost continuously from 1947 to 1960. She is remembered as being 'revered and looked up to' and endeared herself to hundreds of severely injured patients and their families.

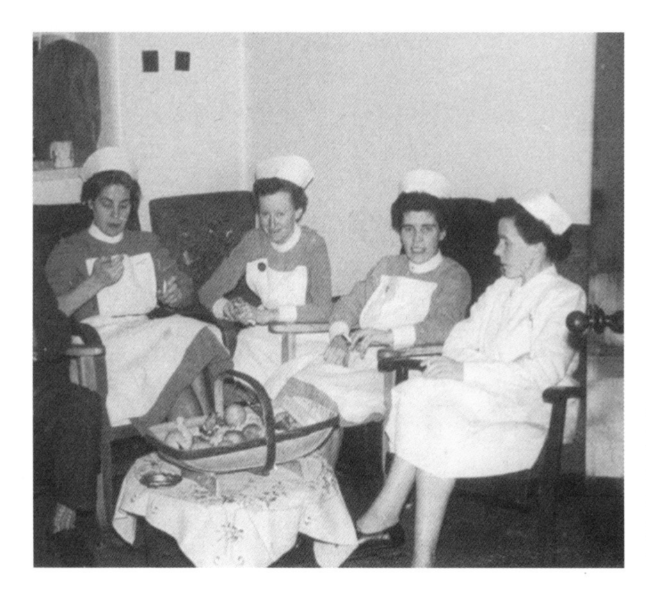

Cronshaw staff relax. From left to right: Barbara Twining, Audrey Driver, Sister Hurley (popularly known as 'Treads' because of the way she said 'threads'' in her Irish accent), -?-.

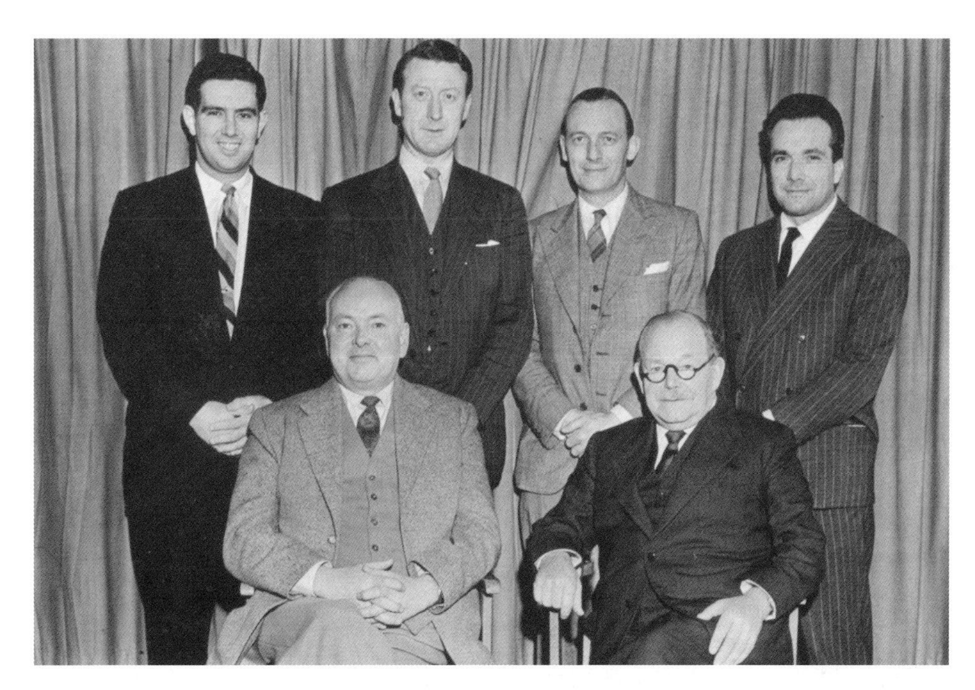

Plastic surgery

The Radcliffe Infirmary was one of the birth places of plastic surgery led by the lively Lancastrian T. Pomfret 'Tommy' Kilner after the First World War when he set up a department which attracted worldwide attention. He became Nuffield Professor of Plastic Surgery in 1944 and was joined in 1946 by Eric Peet who took charge after Kilner retired in 1957. Together they developed surgery for cleft lip and palate and teamed up with Peter Medawar (later Sir Peter), a Nobel Prize-winning scientist doing early work on transplantation.

Here is Tommy Kilner (front right) and Eric Peet (front left) with the Plastic Surgery Department, *c.* 1956.

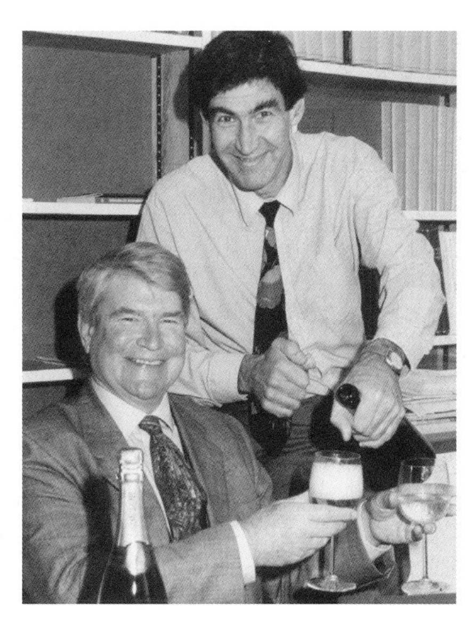

In the 1980s plastic surgeon Michael Poole worked with neurosurgeon Michael Briggs to start what is now the craniofacial service, treating children born with severe skull and facial deformities. Oxford is one of only four craniofacial services in the country and one of nine cleft lip and palate services. Michael Briggs (left) is pictured with Michael Poole.

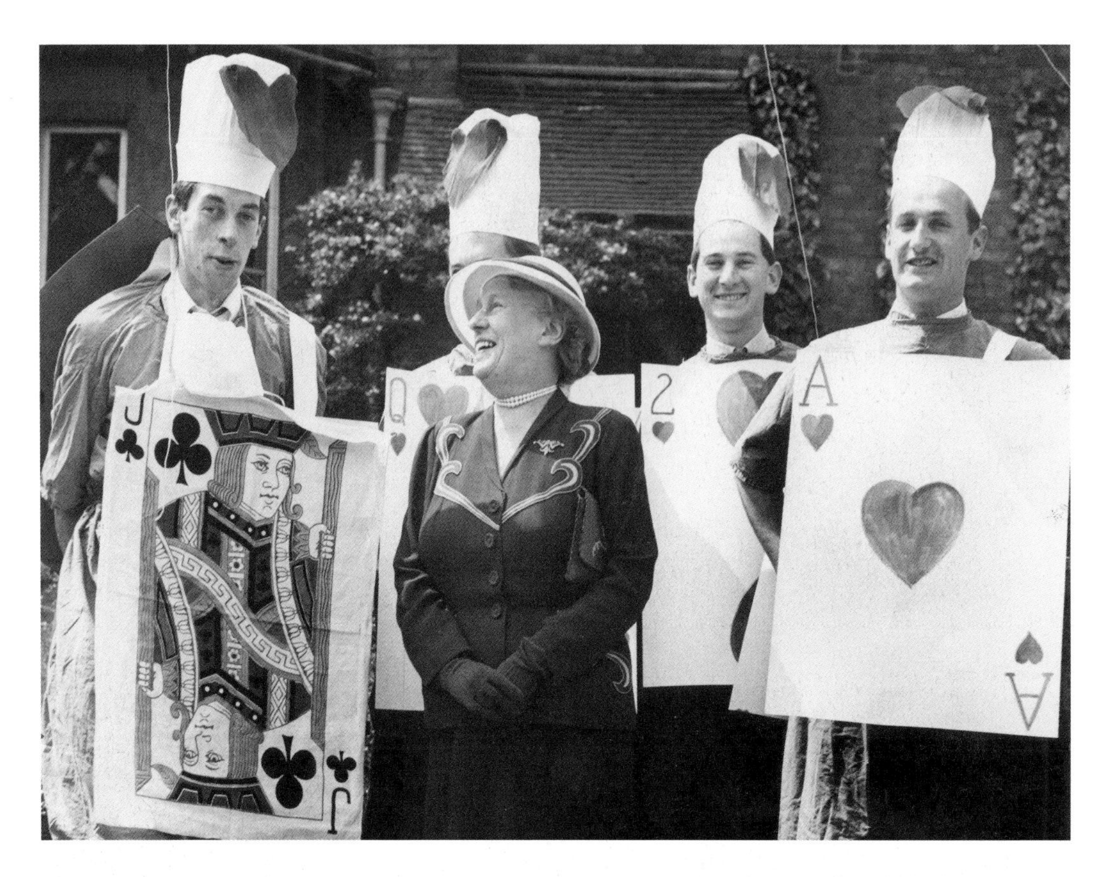

Dermatology

Above: When Dr Alice Carleton, who had led dermatology with, 'lightly worn charm, wit and culture' since 1938, retired in 1957, medical students under a banner 'Alice's Farewell to Wonderland' escorted her from her Banbury Road home to the Infirmary, dressed as playing cards. Among them was Terence Ryan (the ace of hearts), later Professor of Dermatology whose association with the Infirmary as student, doctor, teacher and now historian spans over fifty years.

Dermatology developed more as a significant part of medicine under Renwick Vickers and into a nationally renowned scientific and clinical department under Professor Ryan and Rodney Dawber. (Oxfordshire County Council Photographic Archive – Newsquest)

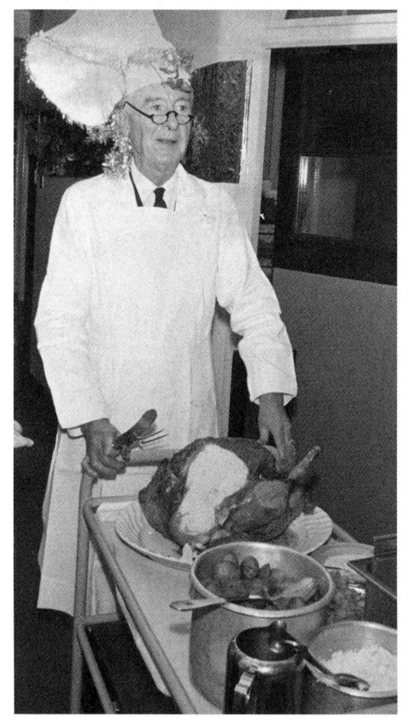

Neurosciences

Right: Neurosurgeon Joe Pennybacker enters into the spirit of Christmas in 1970, carving the turkey on Nuffield ward. Born in Kentucky he studied at Edinburgh and came to Oxford in 1937 as assistant to Hugh Cairns. In 1953 he became director of the Department of Neurosurgery and with John Potter developed a highly regarded service. (Oxfordshire County Council Photographic Archive – Newsquest)

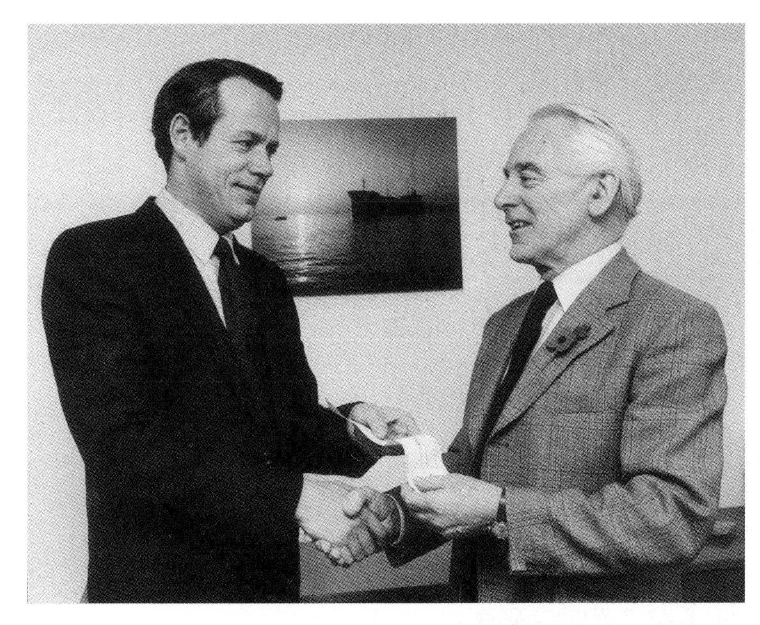

In the latter part of the twentieth century it was Chris Adams (left, receiving a cheque) who took the service forward. In conjunction with neurologist John Oxbury he developed surgery as a successful treatment for some types of epilepsy. (*Oxford Mail and Times*)

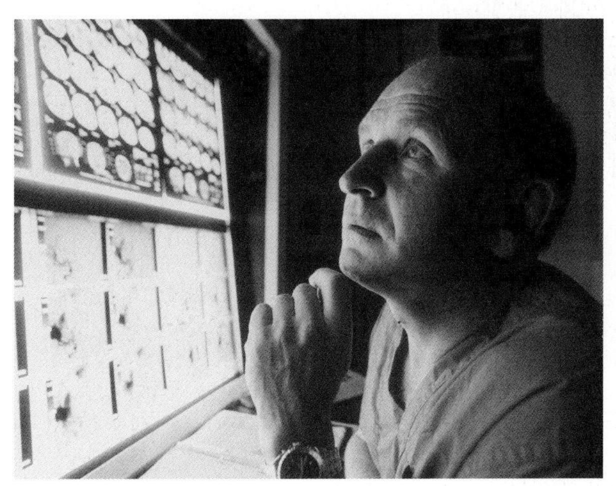

Above: Radiological advances offered alternatives to brain surgery and radiologist Dr Andy Molyneux conducted a major study which compared the outcome for patients who were treated surgically or by interventional radiology. Most patients with an aneurysm are now treated using radiology.

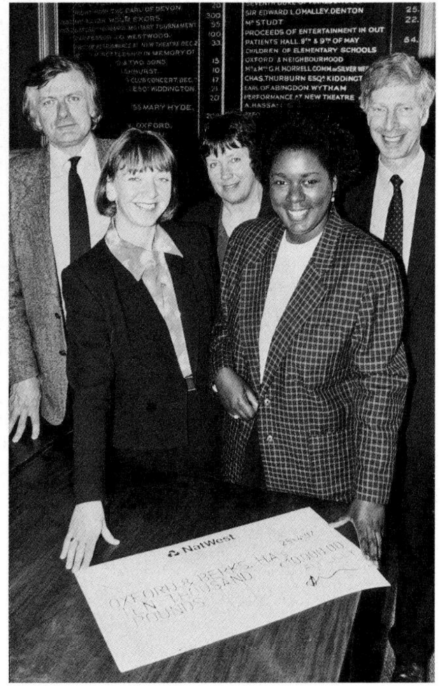

Right: Neurologists, the doctors who see patients when they first come in with symptoms such as seizures, epilepsy, fits, headaches, Parkinson's disease, brain tumour or stroke, and plan the best course of treatment, were also doing pioneering work. Doctors such as Bryan Matthews and John Newsom Davies led the way in services for patients with multiple sclerosis and myasthenia gravis.

A gift from a drug company enabled the Infirmary to have its first specialist nurse for Parkinson's disease patients in 1997. From left to right: Dr Richard Greenhall, Delia Andrew (from Eli Lilly), Anne Scott (senior nurse), Angie Weir (Parkinson's Disease specialist), and Dr Nigel Hyman. (*Oxford Mail and Times*)

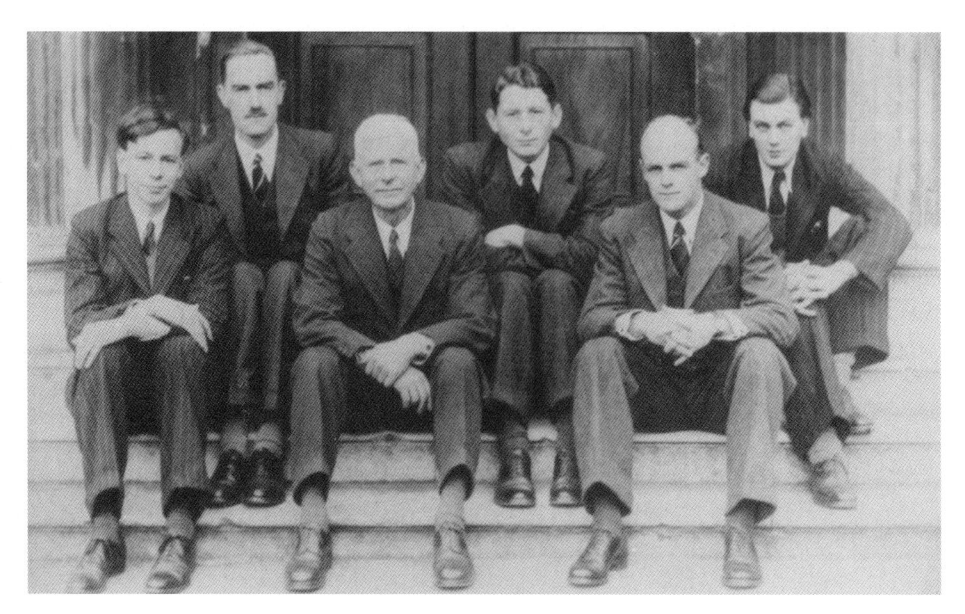

Oxford Medical School

After the war the Goodenough Committee recommended that Oxford University should be given the resources to teach undergraduate medical students. It began with five students in 1948 and reached thirty-two a year by 1950.

This shows the first group of students in October 1948, with the Regius Professor of Medicine A.G. Gardner.

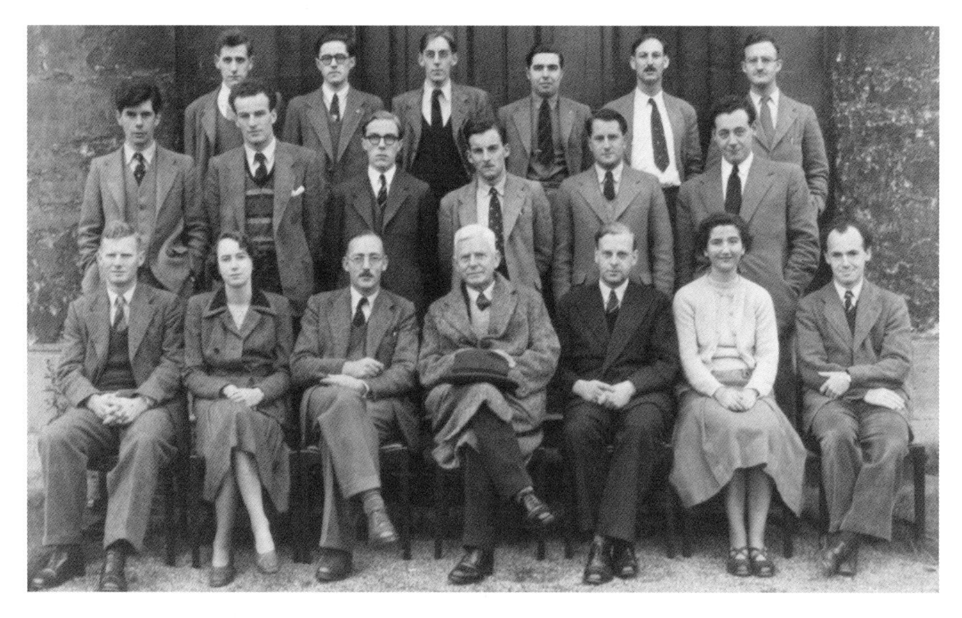

The October 1950 intake, which included some of the first women students. With them (centre left) is Dr Sidney Truelove, a gastroenterologist of originality and distinction, who became director of Clinical Studies in 1949 and in 'a courageous act of realism' wrote a memorandum that analysed the school's progress and argued that it should be developed more fully – which in the ensuing fifty years it has.

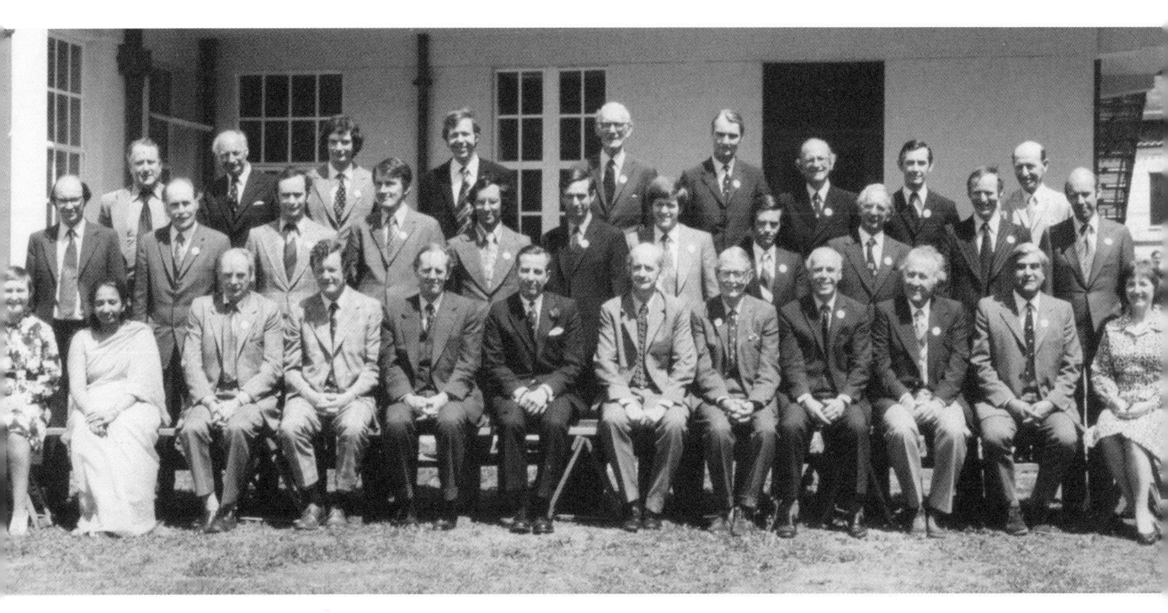

Ear, nose and throat (ENT)

Although there were early pioneers in ear, nose and throat surgery, it was not until 1933 that Ronald Macbeth was appointed the first specialist surgeon.

Within a few years the service was transformed. In 1930 there were 2,500 outpatient attendances and 270 operations. By 1935 there were over 6,000 outpatients and 1,000 operations. Macbeth's career at the Infirmary spanned more than forty years from his student days in the 1920s. He specialised in throats and cancer treatment and was a leading light in the Oxford Caledonian Society.

The picture shows a gathering of leading figures in ear, nose and throat surgery at an international conference in the mid-1970s. Ronald Macbeth is fifth from the right in the front row and Bernard Colman, head of the department, is in the centre. Bill Lund is fifth from the left and Andrew Freeland, at that time recently appointed a consultant, is sixth from the left in the middle row.

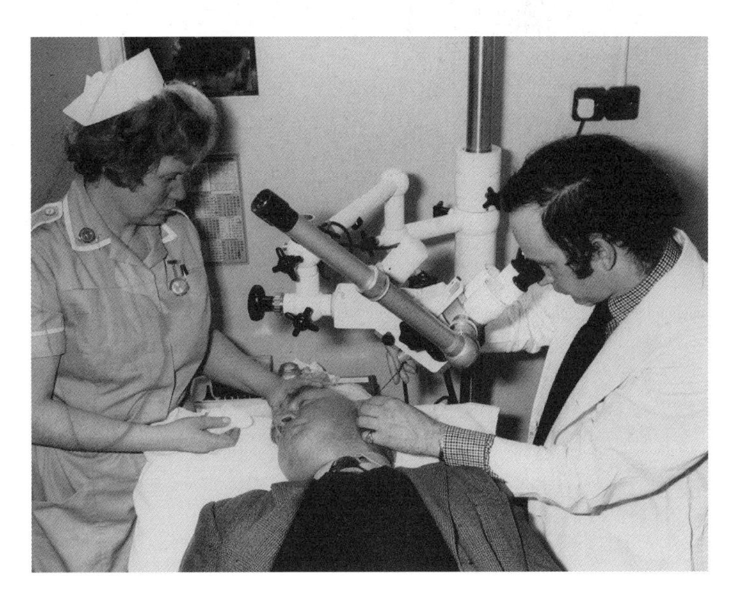

An outpatient examination in the department, *c.* 1975.

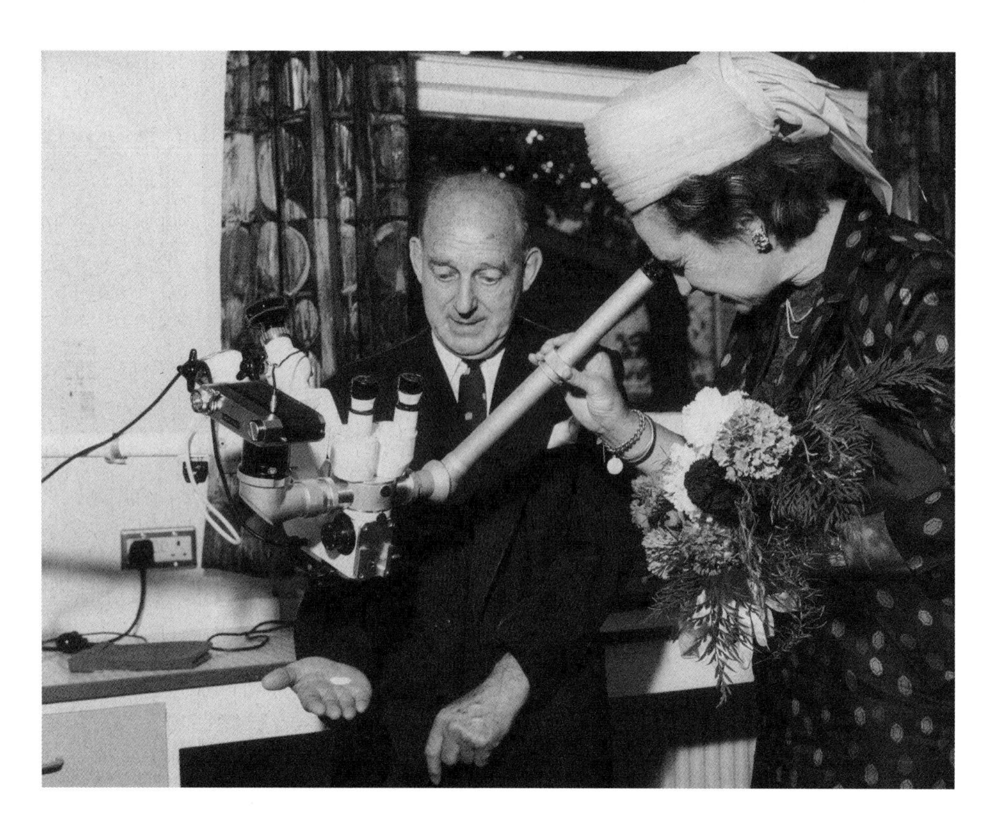

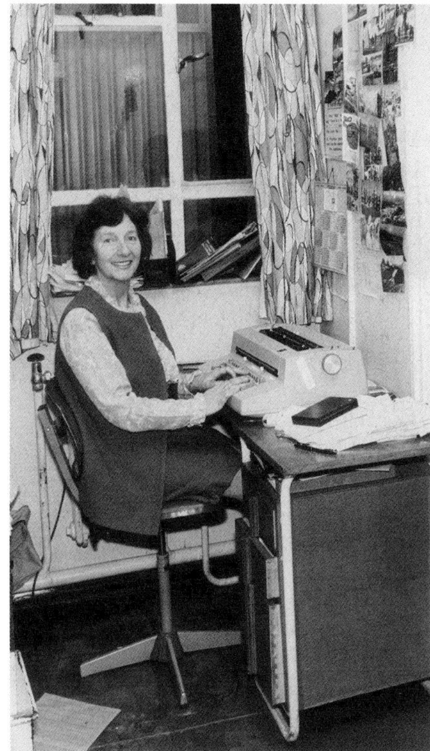

Above: Gavin Livingstone, ENT Surgeon, shows Lady Hoare some equipment at the opening of an annexe to the department in 1967.

Part of the cost was met by the Thalidomide Appeal which had been launched by Lady Hoare five years earlier; children affected by the morning sickness drug often had hearing defects as well as missing or shortened limbs. Gavin Livingstone, who treated many of them, was a surgeon of great skill and gentleness and a man of compassion and unselfishness. He used to throw a party at his home once a year and invite some of the children he had cared for. He died from cancer the year after this picture was taken. (*Oxford Mail and Times*)

Left: Dorothy Scott, 'Scottie' to her contemporaries, worked in the Infirmary for thirty-five years, starting in the Almoner's Department, moving to ENT as a clinical secretary in 1962 and later becoming academic secretary including working on the four-yearly British Academic Conferences in Otolaryngology. She remembers Ronald Macbeth as highly respected and very nice.

Oxford Eye Hospital

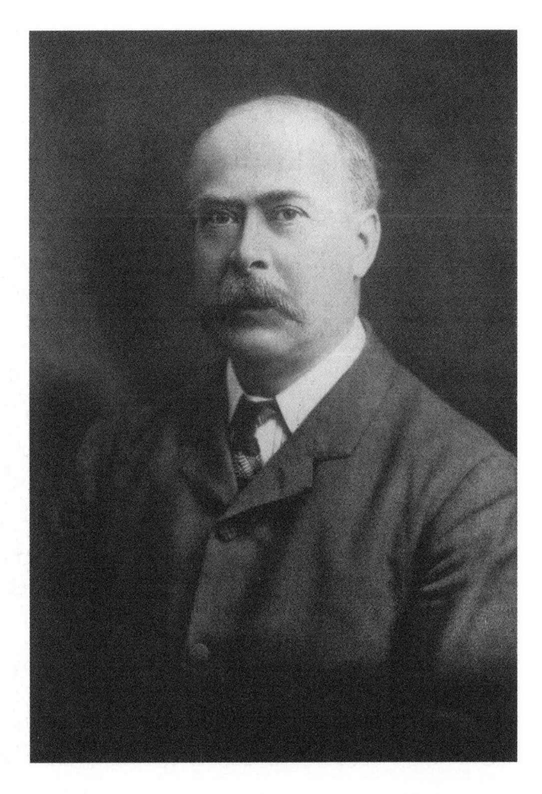

Robert Walter Doyne, the founder of Oxford Eye Hospital. He was a general practitioner with an interest in ophthalmology who saw the need for better eye care and enlisted the help of the mayor and others to establish an eye hospital in 1886, originally in Great Clarendon Street and then in Wellington Square.

It was set up, 'solely for the benefit of the poor' and people paid towards the cost according to their circumstances. Within a short time there were 5,000 attendances a year and more space was needed. In 1894 Doyne leased a building at the Radcliffe Infirmary originally planned as a fever hospital but no longer used as such. With some additions and improvements, the Oxford Eye Hospital occupied the same building until 2006. (Oxford Ophthalmological Congress)

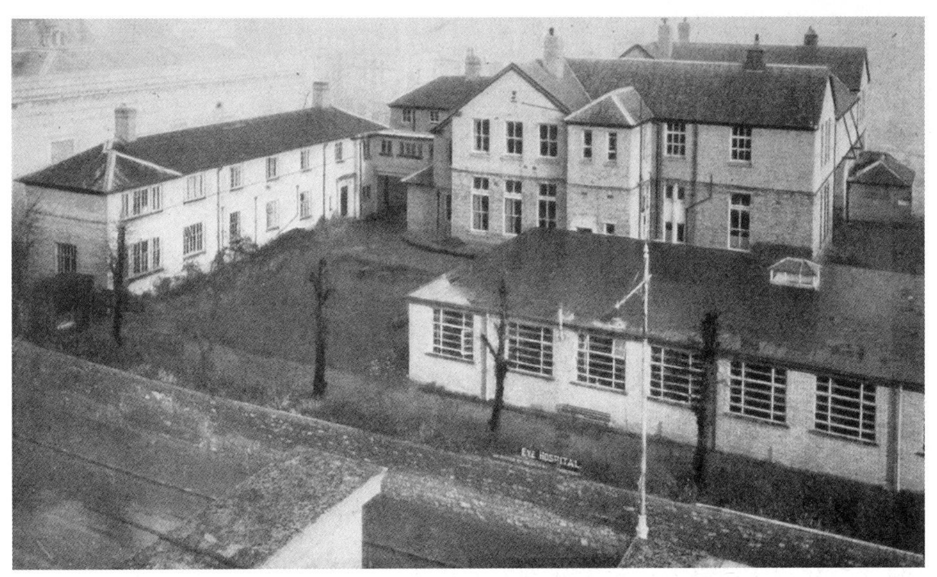

The Eye Hospital in 1945. By now the 1880 fever hospital buildings were, 'wholly inadequate and obsolete' according to an appeal letter issued to raise £100,000 to rebuild them. These pictures come from a booklet produced to show its many drawbacks facing increases in new patients (up from 3,370 to 7,115) and clinic attendances. Forty-one beds were crammed into space for thirty. Despite high powered support, the appeal failed to reach its target, even though it was willing to accept war bonds as an alternative to cash.

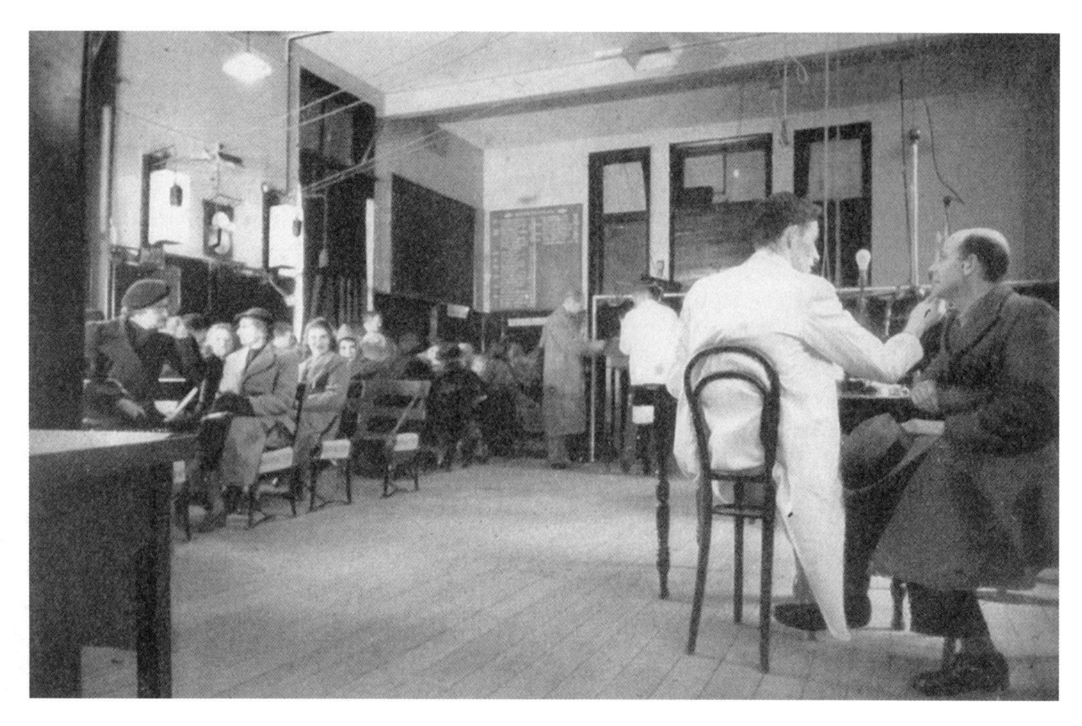

An average of seventy patients plus relatives crowded into this outpatient department to see one of four ophthalmic surgeons engaged in diagnosis and treatments – there was no privacy for consultations.

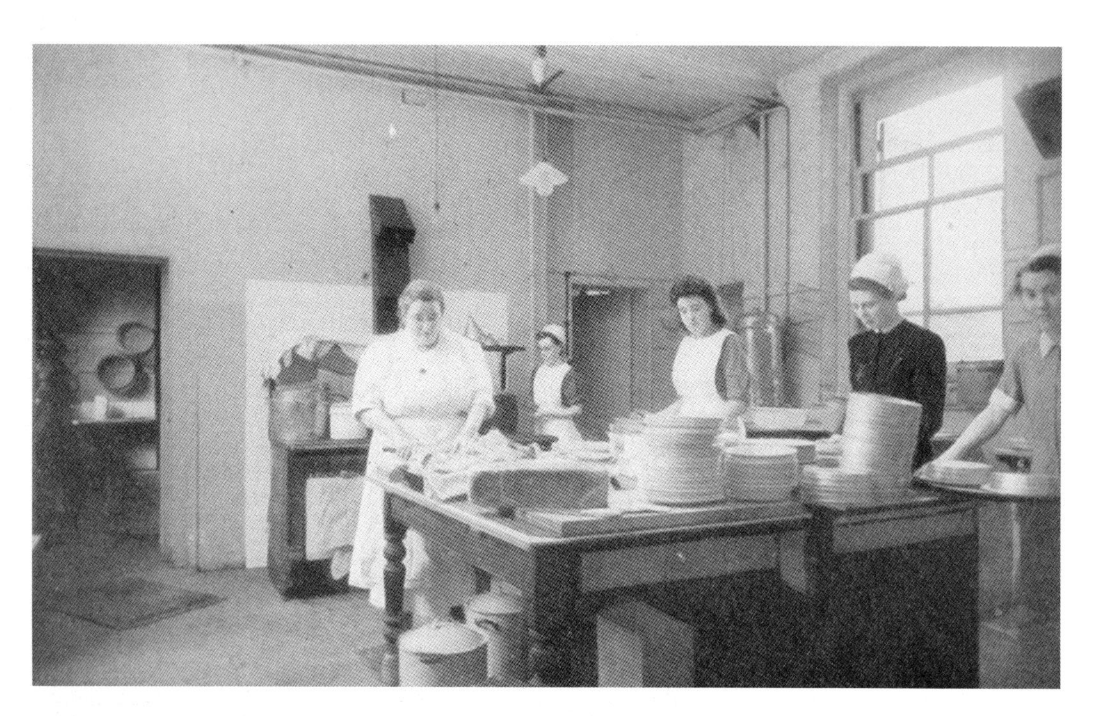

Patient and staff meals were prepared in the kitchen, which had two cupboards and one sink for all purposes.

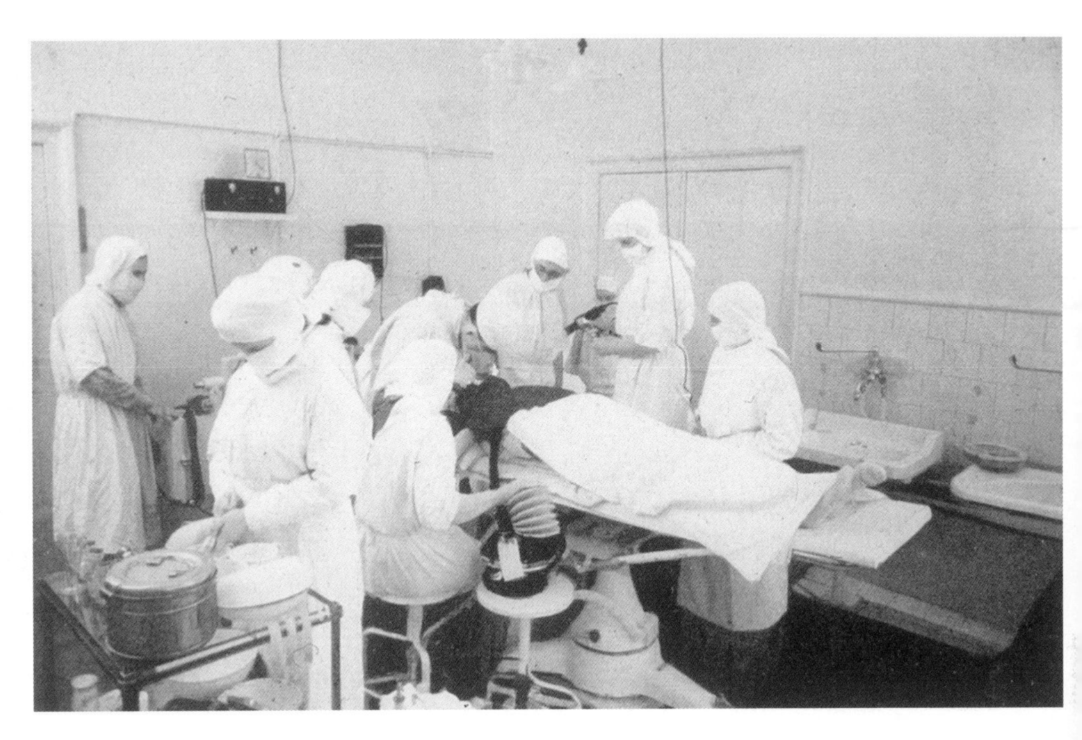

An ante room was converted for use as an operating theatre.

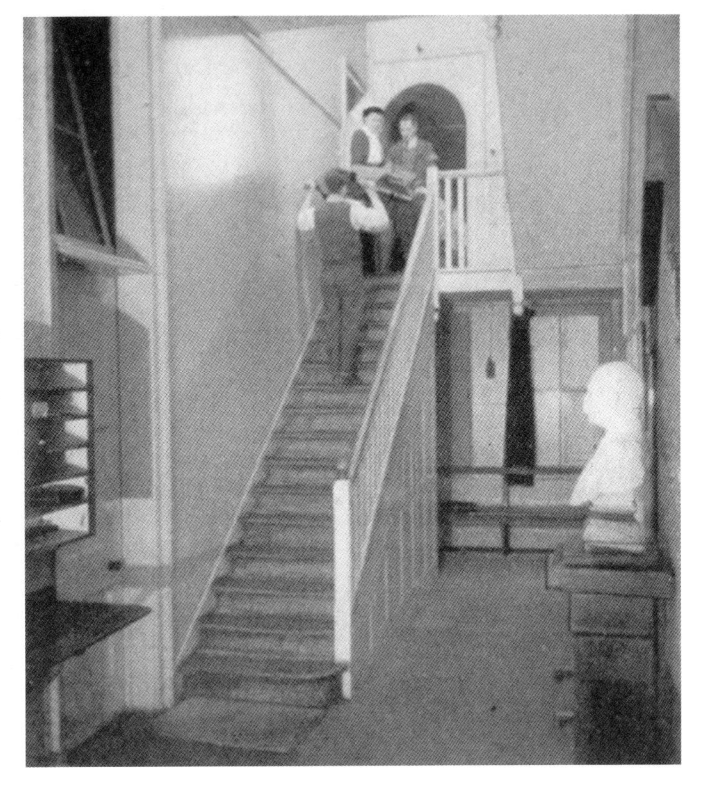

There was no lift so patients on stretchers had to be carried from the ambulance up this flight of stairs and along the corridors to the wards. The stairs are still there, but the inpatient wards moved into the main hospital in 1989-90.

Major alterations were made in 1948 after the fundraising. In 1986 the operating theatres were closed and the surgery transferred to the Towler block. At the end of the twentieth century more than 30,000 patients a year attended outpatient clinics and 13,000 accident and emergency. Optometry and orthoptic clinics together saw more than 20,000 patients.

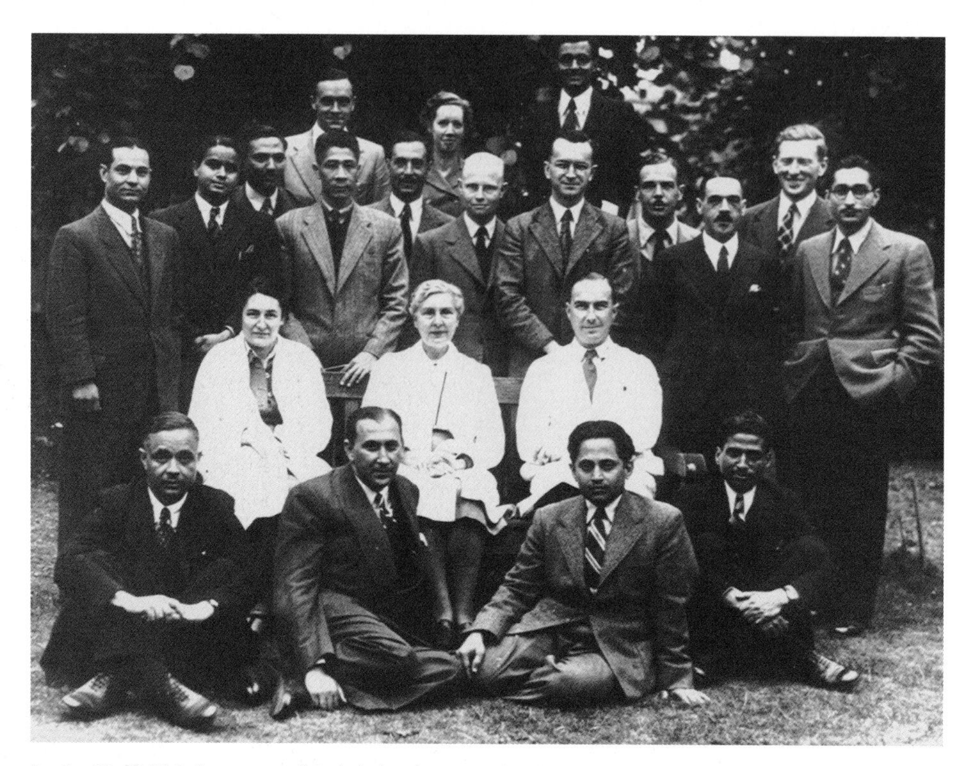

In the Nuffield Laboratory of Ophthalmology nearby, doctors and scientists work closely with the Eye Hospital on research projects. It began with Ida Mann who was appointed reader in Ophthalmology and senior surgeon at Oxford Eye Hospital in 1941 and later became the first woman to hold the title of professor at Oxford. The laboratory was established in 1942 with a gift from Lord Nuffield. This picture of a gathering of staff and visitors around 1950 shows Ida Mann (centre) and her successor as head of the department, Antoinette Pirie, on her right.

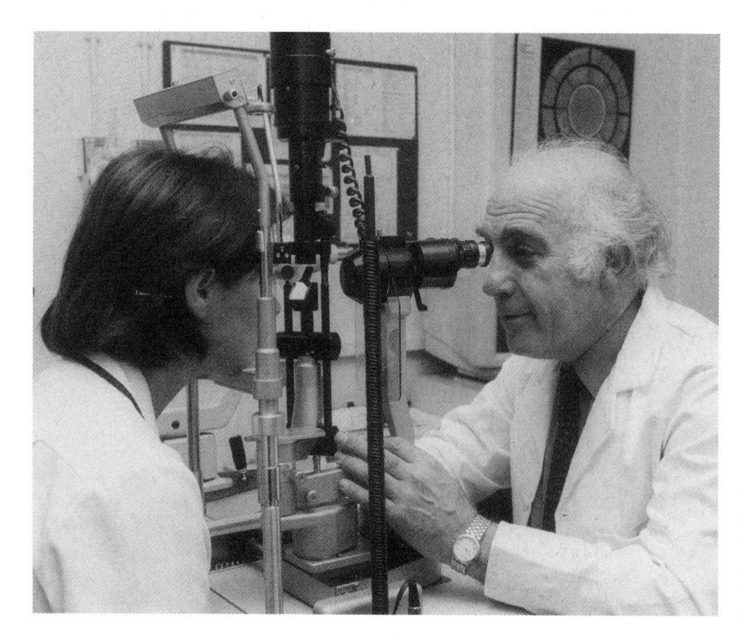

A modern service in an old building. Professor Anthony Bron conducts an eye examination in 1999.

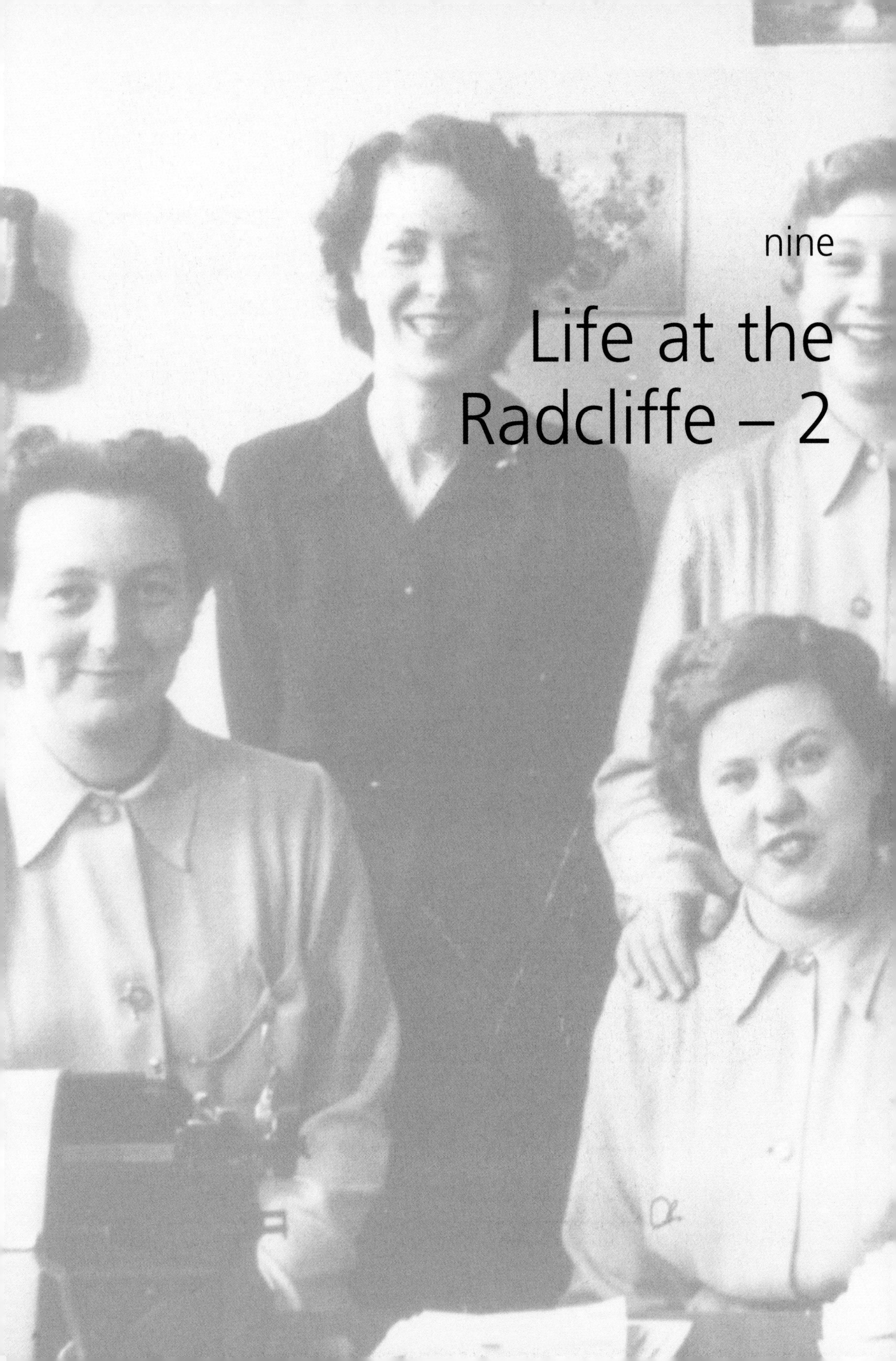

nine

Life at the Radcliffe – 2

A student's life in the late 1950s. These pictures from Francois Retief, who later became director-general of National Health and vice-chancellor of the University of the Orange Free State, record his days as a medical student at Oxford.

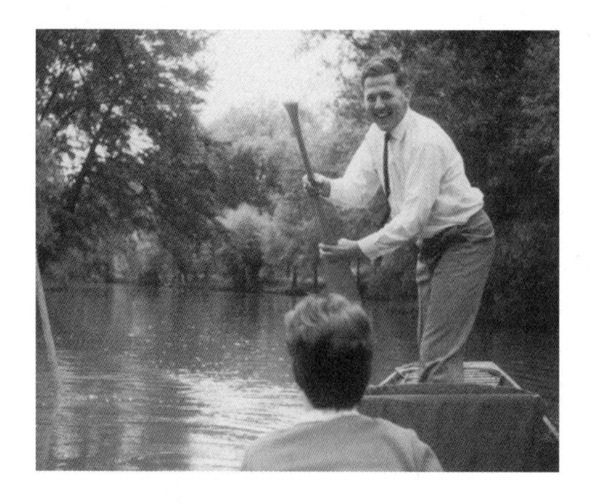

Left: Punting on the Cherwell – having left the pole in the mud.

Below left: Skating on Port Meadow.

Below right: Medical staff *v.* students rugby, 1957.

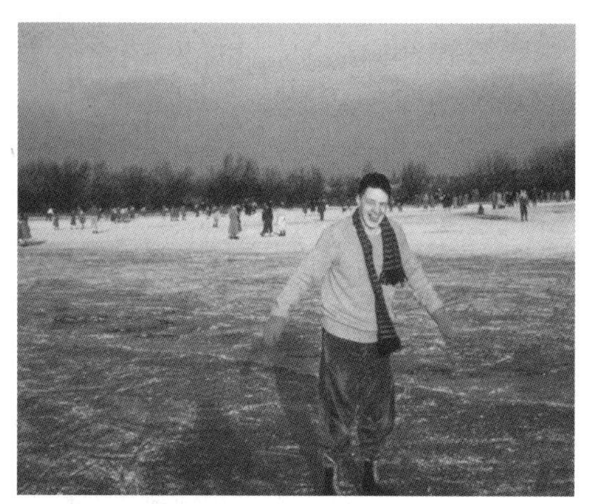

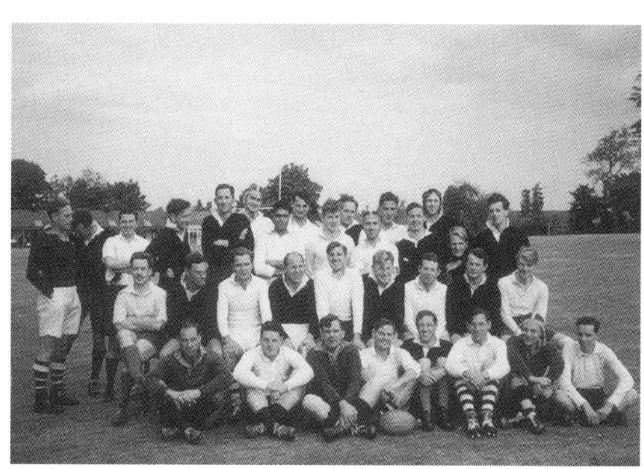

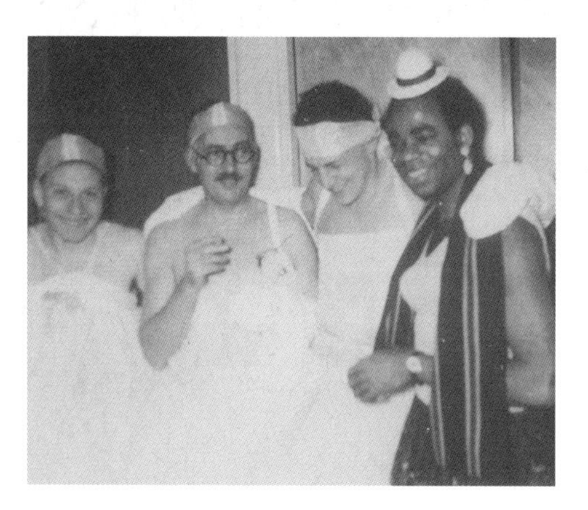

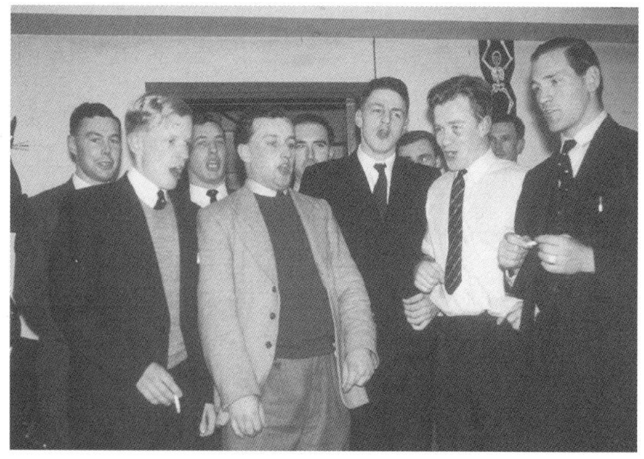

Above left: Fairies in the pantomime in 1958, with M. Raphael, Sidney Truelove and Fidelis Uden.

Above right: Last night in Osler House, 1959.

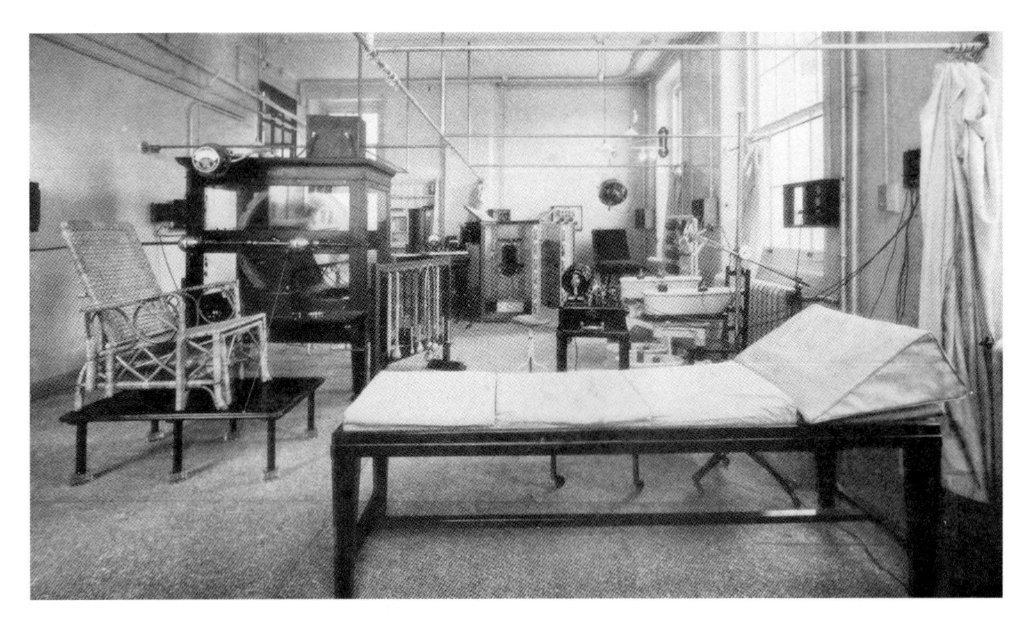

Physiotherapy

The electrotherapeutic department in 1913. Dr Walter Turrell was appointed 'electrotherapeutic physician' in 1908 and revolutionised physiotherapy, leading the way in the use of electricity for something other than shock treatment. His department was full of apparatus, often homemade, and he was ably supported by a team of masseuses and assistants. When he retired in 1938 he was an international authority on physiotherapy.

Right: A 'static bicycle' being used to regain power in the legs after polio in 1959. At that time the hospital had two doctors, twelve physiotherapists and two occupational therapists carrying out between 7,000 and 8,000 treatments a month in the rapidly growing field of 'physical medicine'. (*Oxford Mail and Times*)

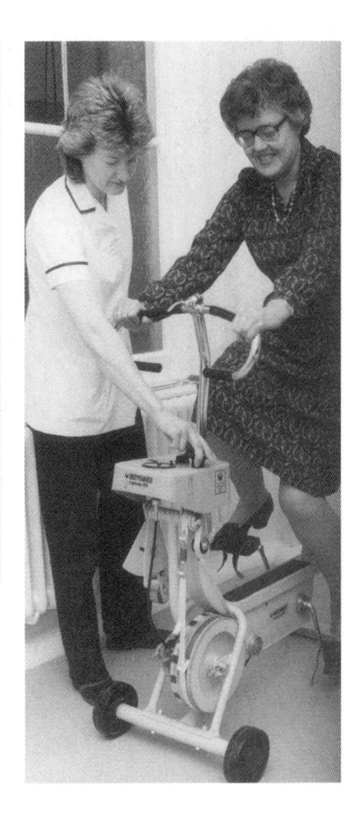

Far right: Physiotherapy moved to new premises on the ground floor in 1987 to provide more space and give easier access for patients. About 1,300 patients a month were treated there. Mrs Caroline Miles, chairman of Oxfordshire Health Authority, opened the department and tried an exercise bike, watched by superintendent physiotherapist Mary Lightbody. (*Oxford Mail and Times*)

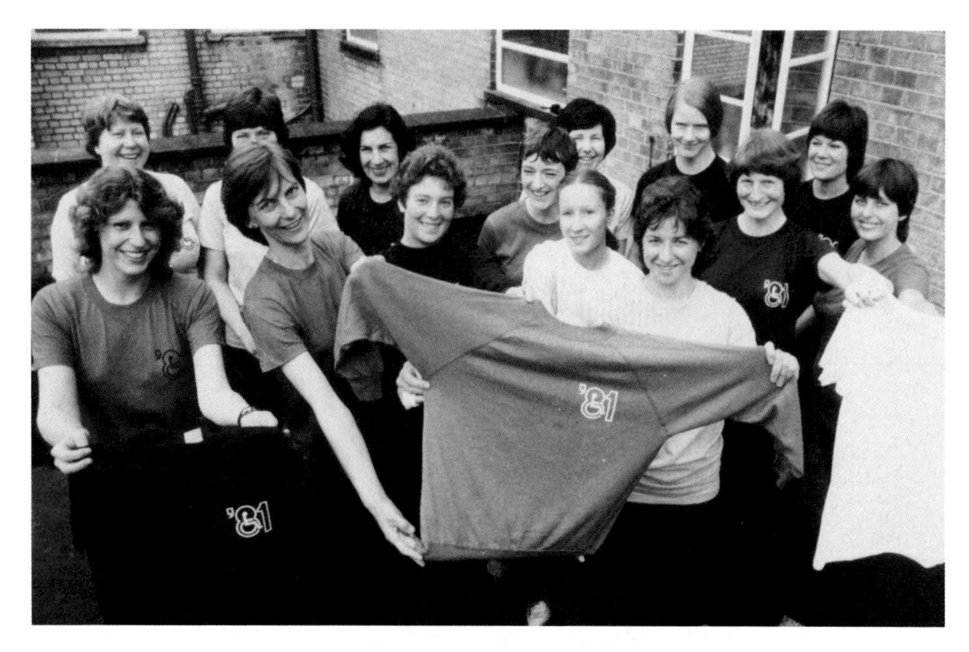

Physiotherapy staff in 1981 with special shirts and tops for the Year of the Disabled.

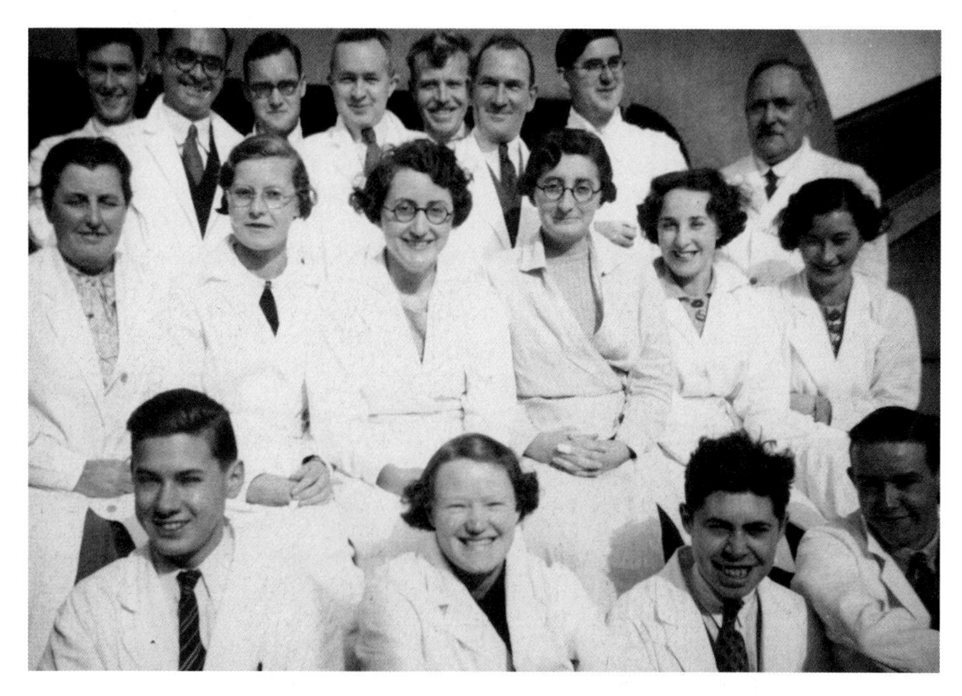

Staff from the Departments of Biochemistry and Pathology, 1938. Amos Chown, the redoubtable chief technician who began work as a lab boy at the age of fourteen in 1905, is in the back row, third from right. He was an invaluable member of the department and undertook many extra duties such as taking blood from patients. He took charge of generations of technicians. Robb-Smith (second right, back row) recalls his, 'kindly equanimity'. Technicians recall a strict disciplinarian, especially with regard to punctuality.

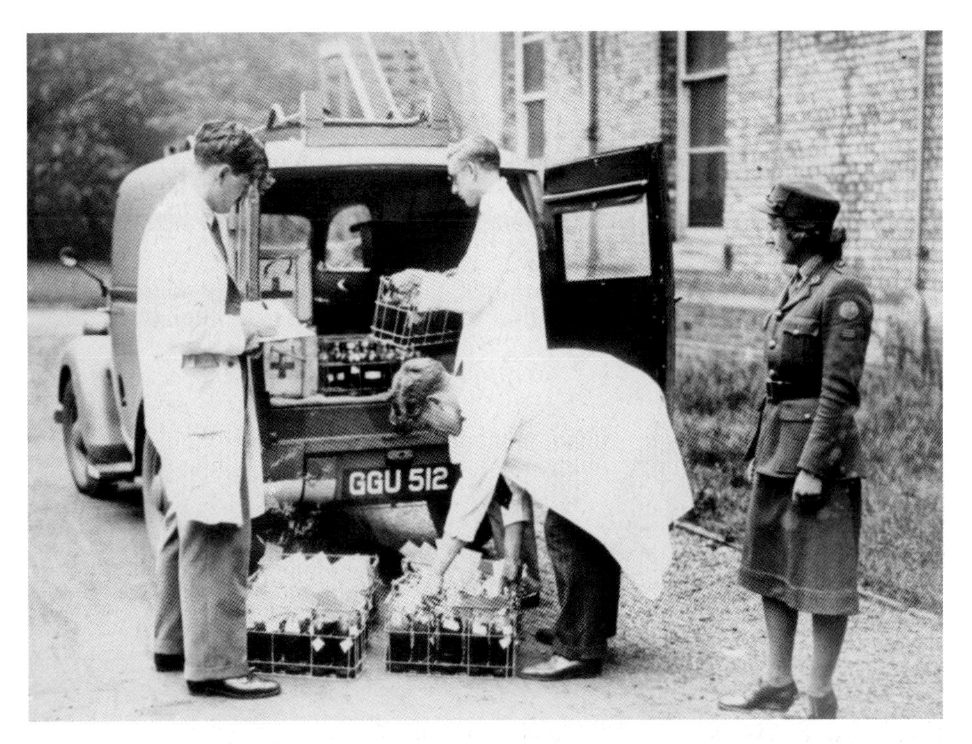

Dr W. Ormorod, John Morton and M.J. Allington unload blood collected from donors in the new Bodleian Library during the Second World War. The wartime blood transfusion service was largely run by volunteers with the help of doctors from the Infirmary and provided about 3,000 bottles of blood and plasma a year for local civilian and military hospitals. In June and July 1944 they collected 2,000 bottles of blood in anticipation of invasion casualties.

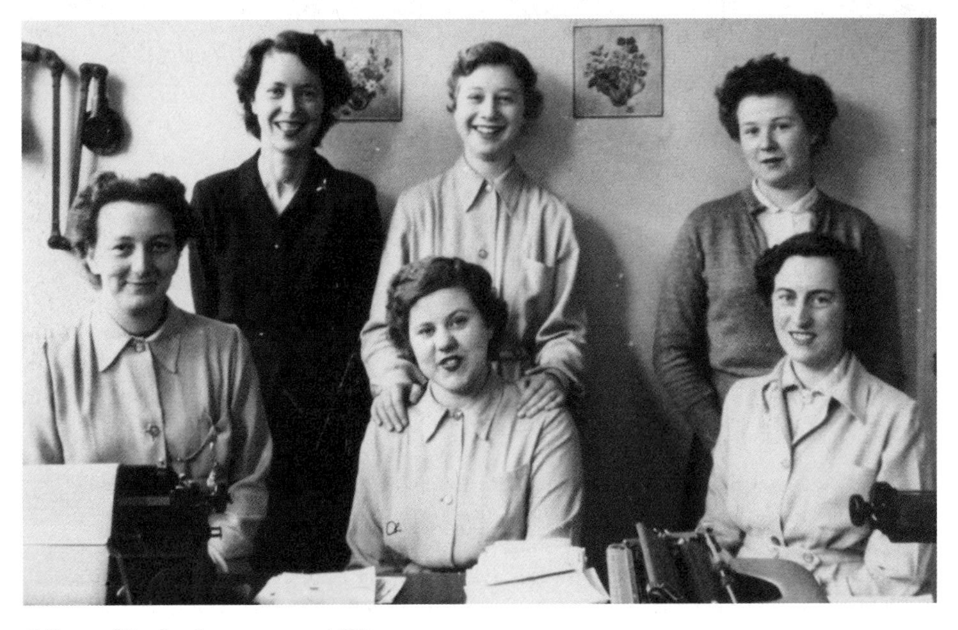

Office staff in the department, *c.* 1955.

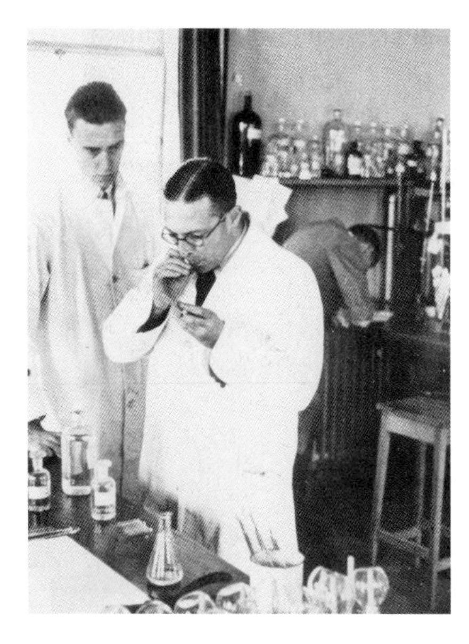

Dr J.R.P. O'Brien, director of the Department of Biochemistry, at work in the laboratory around 1952, watched by Ken Scholes.

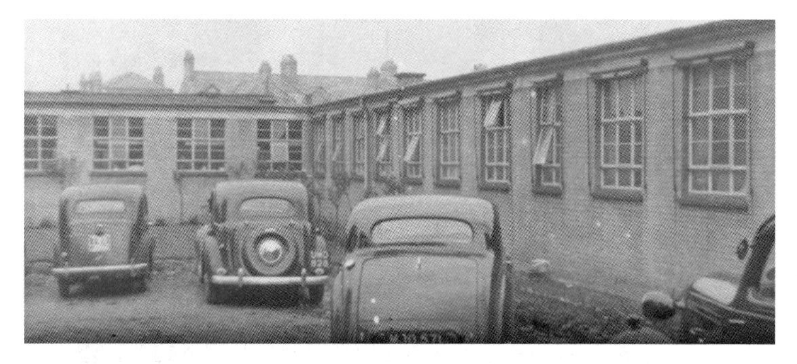

Departments of Haematology and Blood Transfusion, Bacteriology and Public Health Bacteriology buildings, *c.* 1952. The departments opened in 1945.

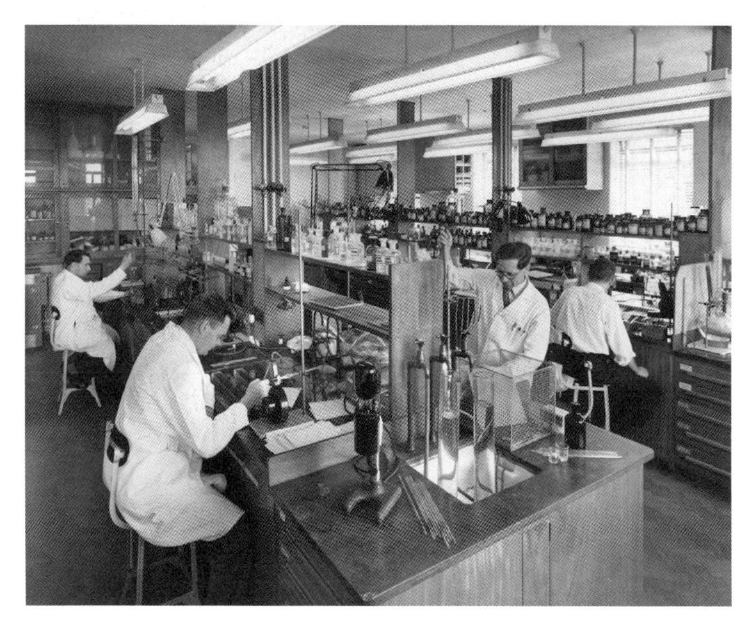

Radcliffe Infirmary Laboratories, *c.* 1970.

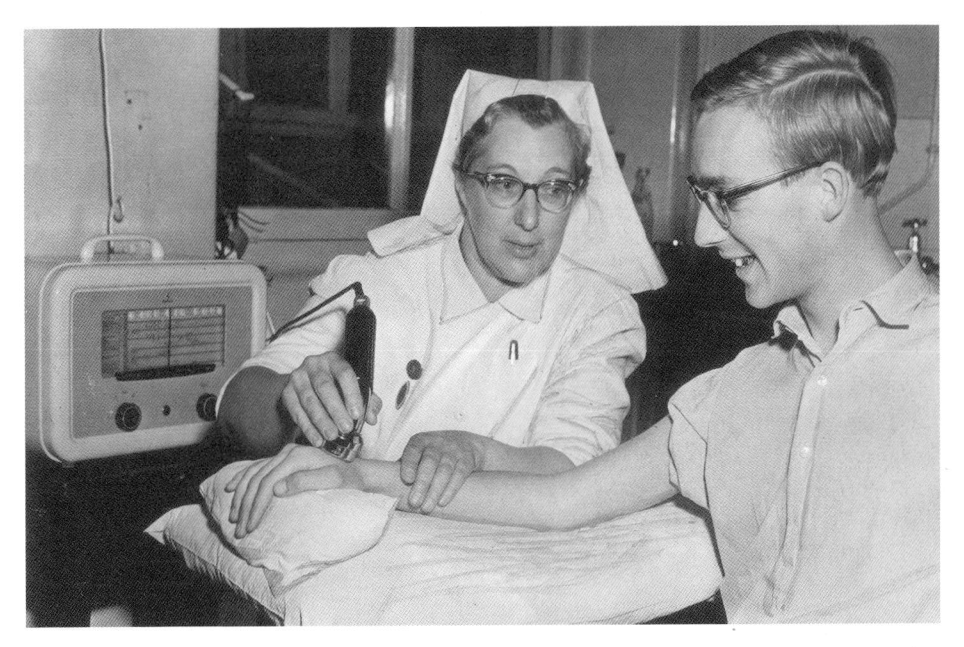

The use of ultrasound to treat injuries is commonplace now, but in the 1950s it was still relatively new. This picture from 1959 depicts, 'the most recent form of treatment – ultrasonics – being applied to a disabled hand'. (*Oxford Mail and Times*)

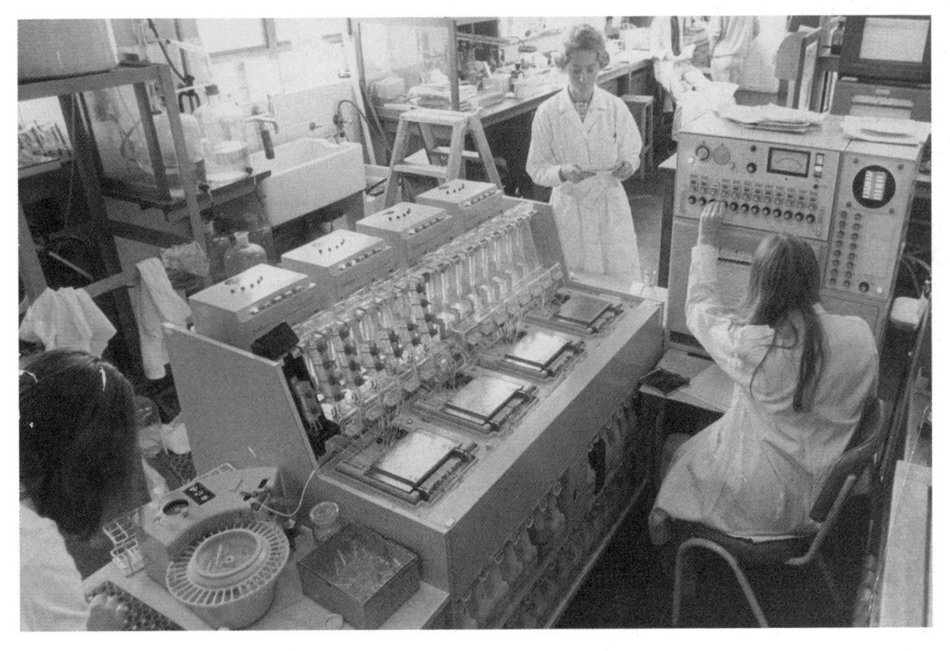

The development of laboratory services – and the speed at which tests could be done – was one of the features of the later years of the twentieth century. Here the hospital was proud to show off, 'one of the most up to date aids in diagnostic work in the biochemistry laboratory', a £20,000 blood analyser which could do twelve tests on a blood sample in a minute. The results were printed in red ink on paper. (*Oxford Mail and Times*)

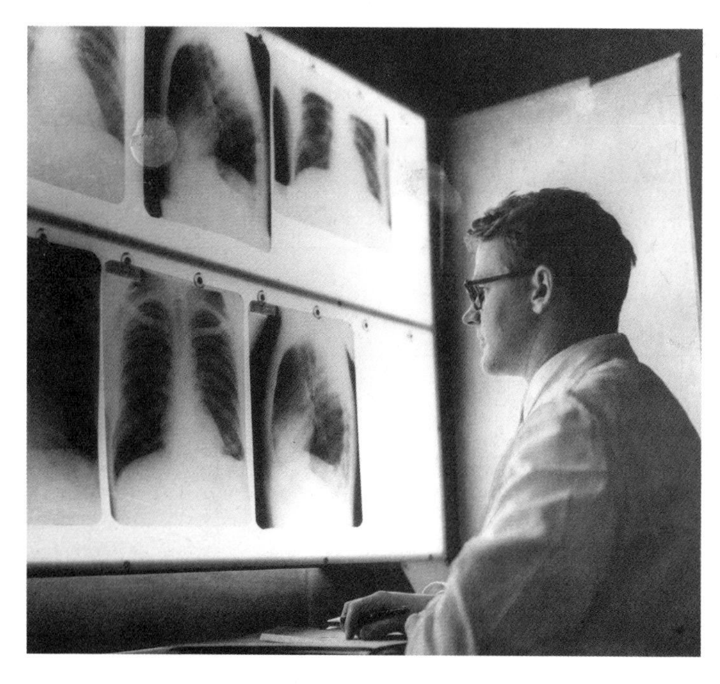

Examining X-rays, *c.* 1959. X-rays were first used at the Infirmary before the First World War when Dr R.H. Sankey was appointed 'radiographer' and started the department in a hut near the operating theatre. In 1933 the service moved into a properly designed department. Sankey intended to retire in 1939 but was persuaded to continue until 1945. (*Oxford Mail and Times*)

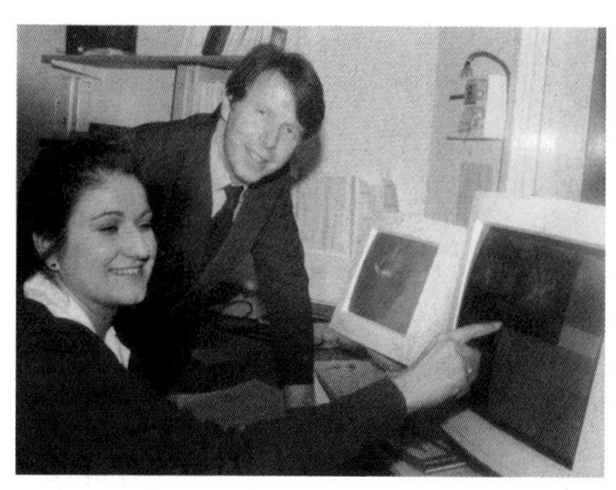

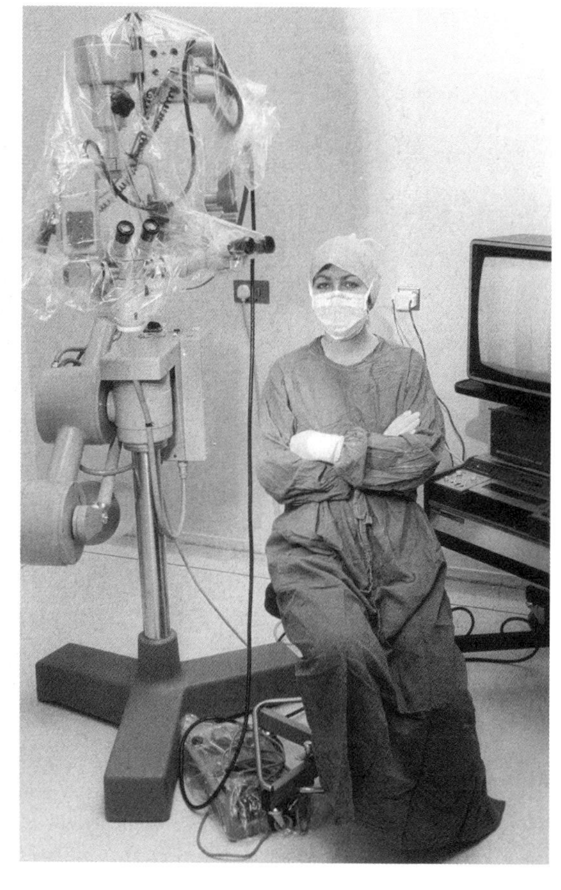

Right: Major advances in the use of microscopes in surgery – microsurgery – took place in the 1970s and 1980s. At the Infirmary neurosurgeons, plastic surgeons, eye surgeons and ENT surgeons were soon using equipment like this £15,000 microscope which in 1980 was the only one of its kind in the country. (*Oxford Mail and Times*)

Above: Move on to another decade and it's Magnetic Resonance Imaging (MRI) which is the new diagnostic tool of the 1990s. Minister for Health Tom Sackville is with senior radiographer Virginia Moody when he opened a new scanner in 1994. (*Oxford Mail and Times*)

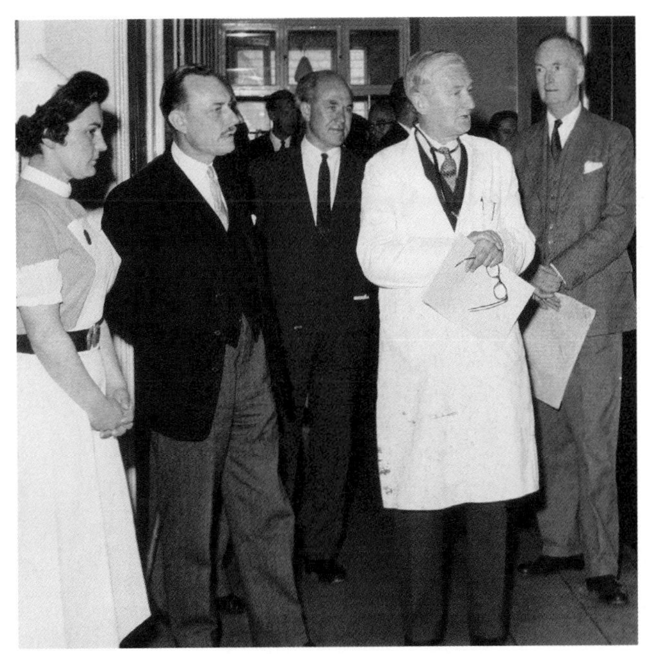

Enoch Powell, Minister for Health, visited the Radcliffe Infirmary in May 1961. He is seen here with Professor Leslie Witts, Nuffield Professor of Clinical Medicine (in white coat) and Sir Oliver (later Lord) Franks, chairman of the Board of Governors of United Oxford Hospitals. Looking on left is Miss J. King, Sister of Willis ward, a female ward in the Nuffield Department of Medicine, which opened in 1957.

Professor Witts was appointed the first Nuffield Professor of Medicine at Oxford in 1937. He had a special interest in blood disorders but also a wide interest in general medicine and its psychological aspects. It was said that there were professors all over the world who had sat at his feet in Oxford. The Witts lecture theatre at the Infirmary was named after him. (*Oxford Mail and Times*)

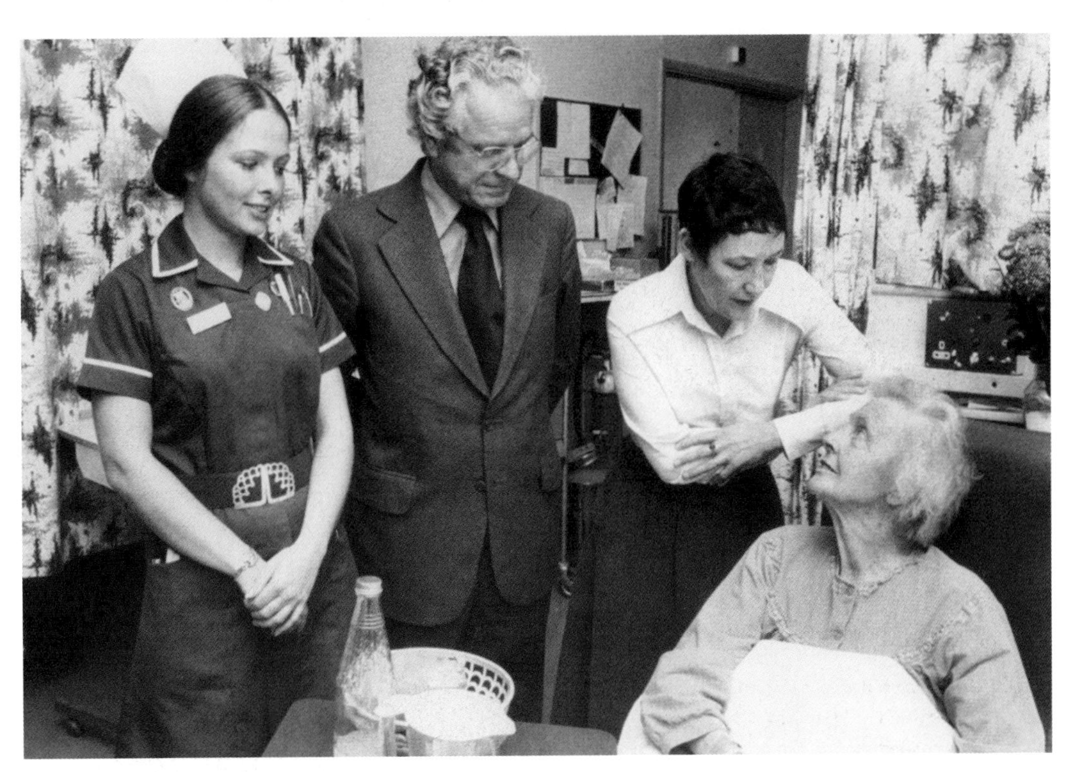

The dedication of staff who were working to high standards in overcrowded and unsuitable conditions was praised by the new chairman of Oxford Regional Health Authority Gordon Roberts (later Sir Gordon) when he visited in 1978 at the start of a tour of hospitals in the region. With him is Lady McCarthy, chairman of Oxfordshire Area Health Authority, and Sister Elizabeth Sims. (*Oxford Mail and Times*)

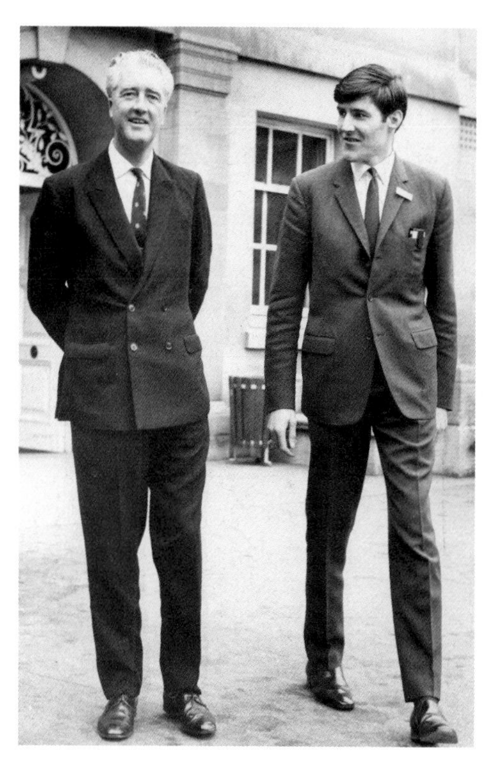

Left: Lord Aberdare, Minister of State at the Department of Heath and Social Security (left) visited the Radcliffe in October 1970 for talks about new styles of management at United Oxford Hospitals. He is seen here with Robin Lawson, house governor.

The Infirmary was often an innovator in management practice as well as clinical practice. It was the first provincial hospital to have an admissions office and it piloted developments in electronic supplies ordering in the 1980s and resource management in the 1990s. (Oxfordshire County Council Photographic Archive – Newsquest)

Below: When the Infirmary celebrated its 200th anniversary in 1970 it began celebrations with a 'thank you' reception for staff representatives and supporters at Oxford Town Hall. Church services took place on the actual date and there was a ball at Blenheim Palace, concerts and an exhibition. Seen here at the Town Hall reception are Sister M. Flemming being greeted by one of the governors, Mr Les Davies, watched by Mr H.H. Johnston and Professor Ritchie Russell. (*Oxford Mail and Times*)

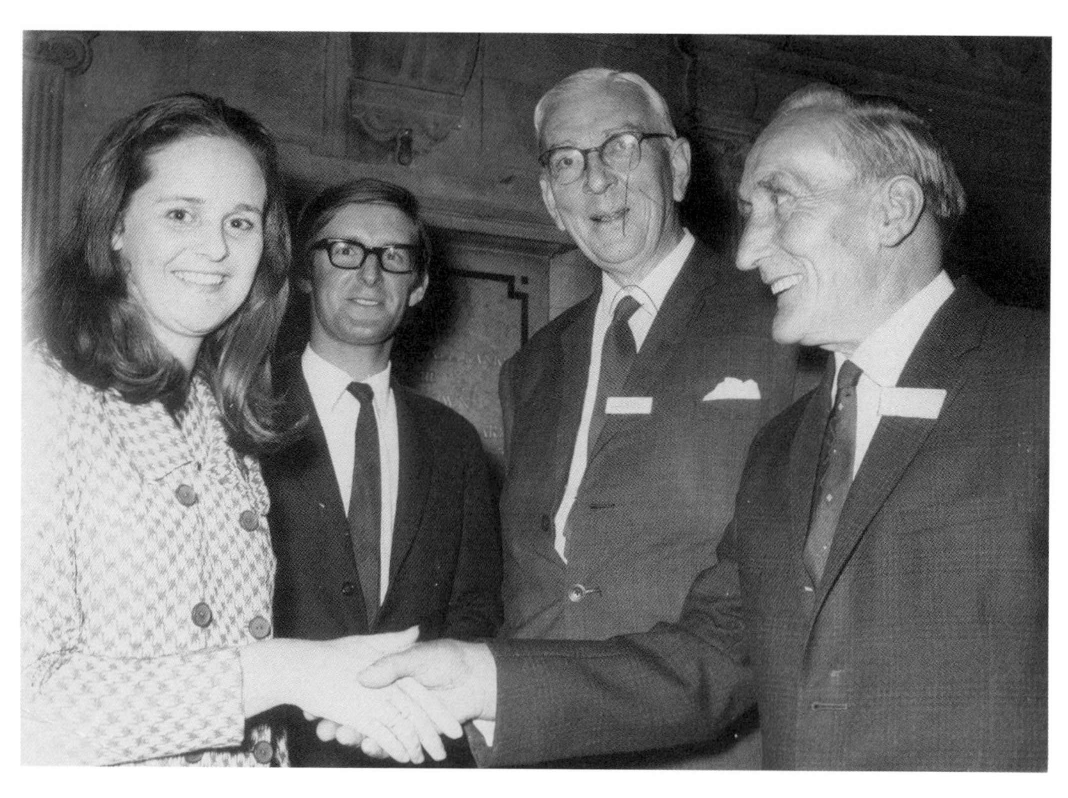

Lord Rosenheim, president of the Royal College of Physicians, plants a tree in 1970. With him, from left to right, are: Dr Alastair Robb-Smith, Professor (later Sir Richard) Doll and Alan Bullock, vice-chancellor of the university. The tree was from a seed of a tree in Kos under which Hippocrates was said to have administered. Sir Richard Doll's pioneering studies proved conclusively that smoking caused lung cancer and other illnesses. (*Oxford Mail and Times*)

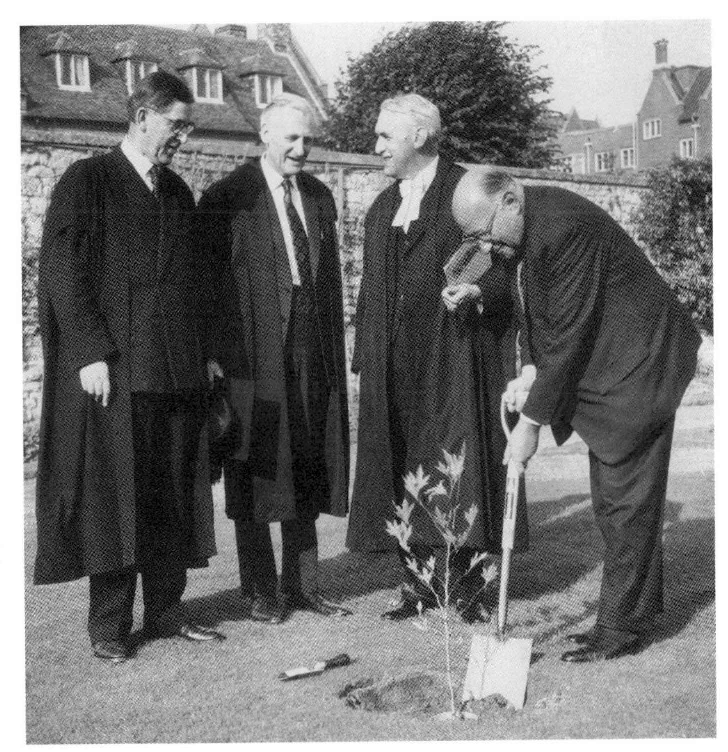

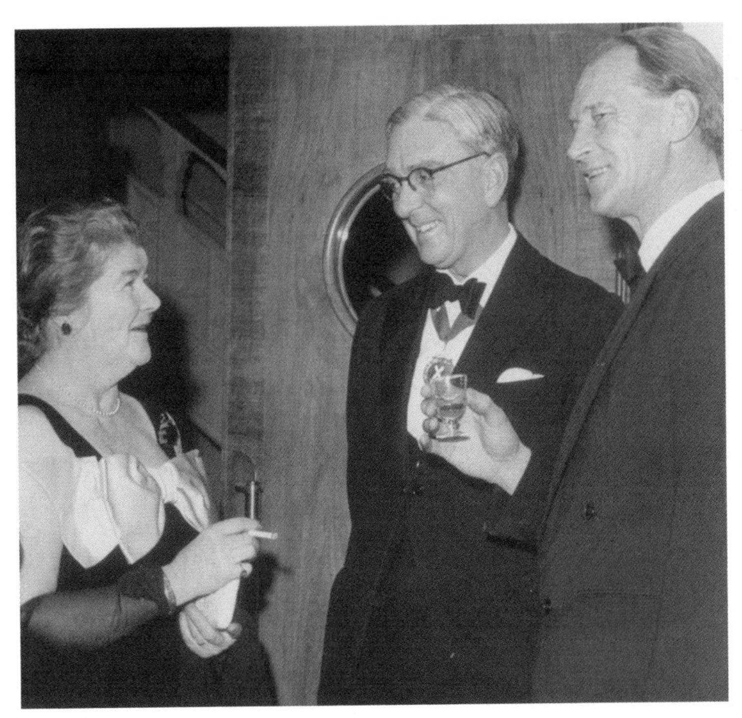

Professor Ritchie Russell with guests E.J.R. Burrough and Mrs Burrough at an Oxford event. Ritchie Russell was honorary consultant neurologist to the army during the war and returned to create one of the largest departments of academic neurology in the country. He led research which compiled an index of thousands of people with severe brain injury and then followed up their progress. In later years he did important work on behalf of people with brain damage.

E.J.R. 'Jum' Burrough was administrator for United Oxford Hospitals from 1951 to 1969 and author of *Unity in Diversity*, the history of United Oxford Hospitals. (*Oxford Mail and Times*)

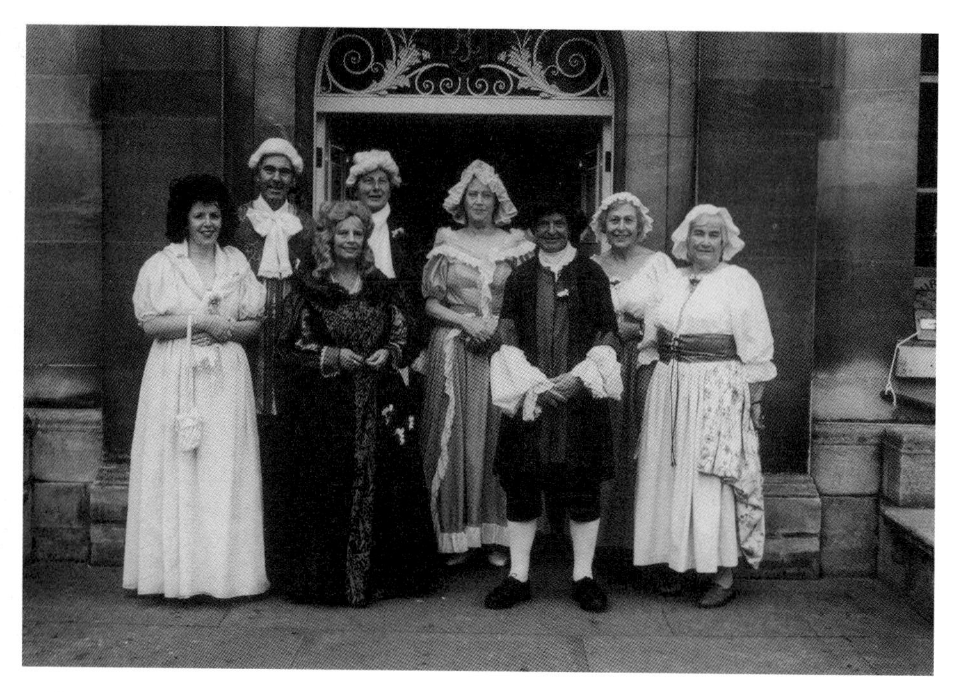

Staff in period costume for the celebrations when the hospital was 225 years old in 1995.

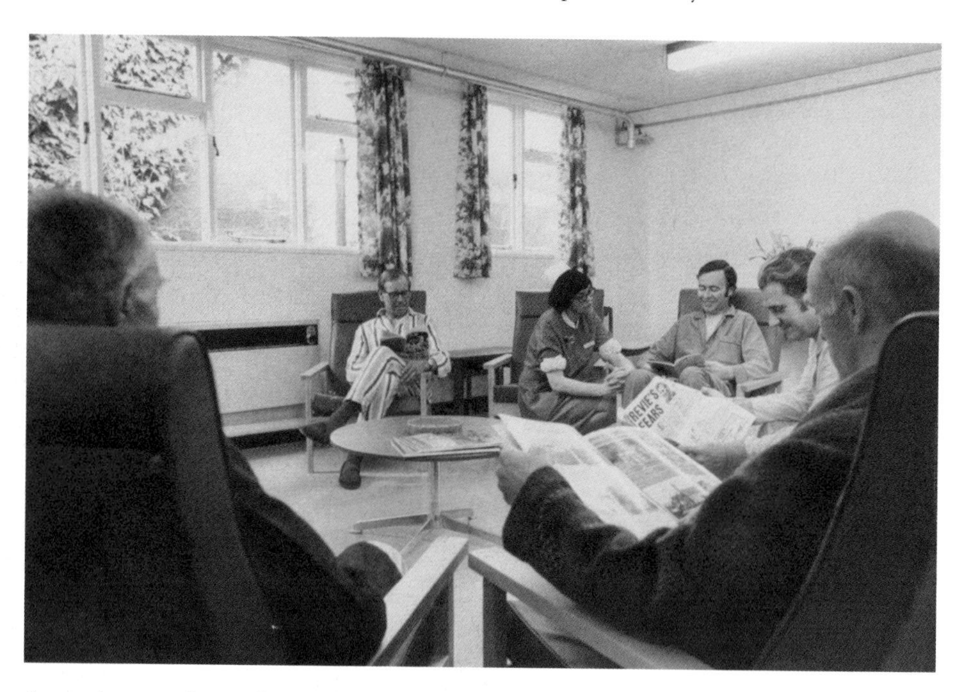

A new day room for Marlborough ward opened in 1975, converted from an old storage hut. It was paid for by the Oxford Hospitals Services Development Fund and furnished by the League of Friends. The fund was a descendant of Dr William Collier's 2*d* a week contributory scheme from the 1920s. Thousands of people – many of them workers in factories and offices around Oxford – contributed small amounts from their pay packet each week. (*Oxford Mail and Times*)

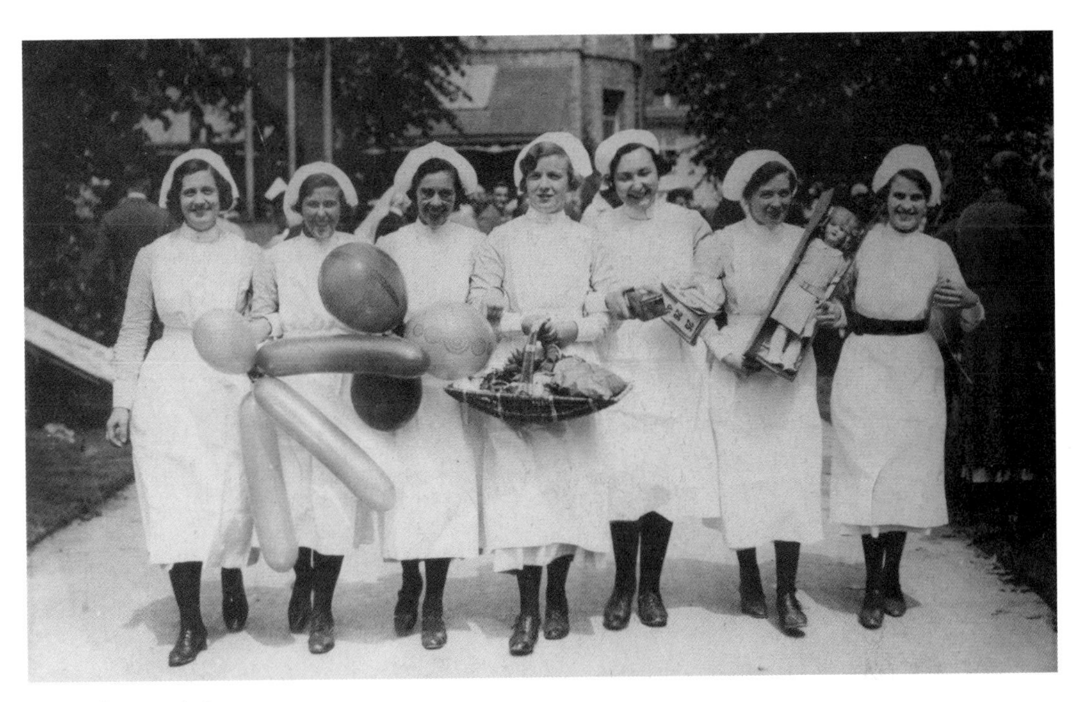

The social scene

Nurses taking part in the 1933 hospital fête with collecting box, raffle tickets and prizes in hand. Hospital staff were frequently involved in fundraising and social events and members of the public and local organisations were regular visitors bringing cheques and gifts. Staff often took part in 'fun' events. Father Christmas was a regular visitor to the wards and the famous Christmas pantomime – 'Tynchwycke' – was a popular tradition for decades.

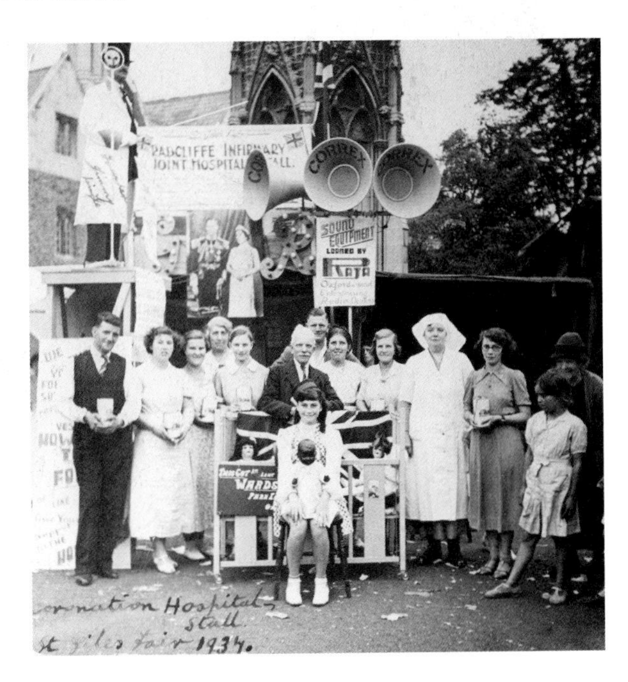

Staff at the 'Coronation' hospital stall at St Giles' Fair in 1937, with the Martyrs Memorial in the background.

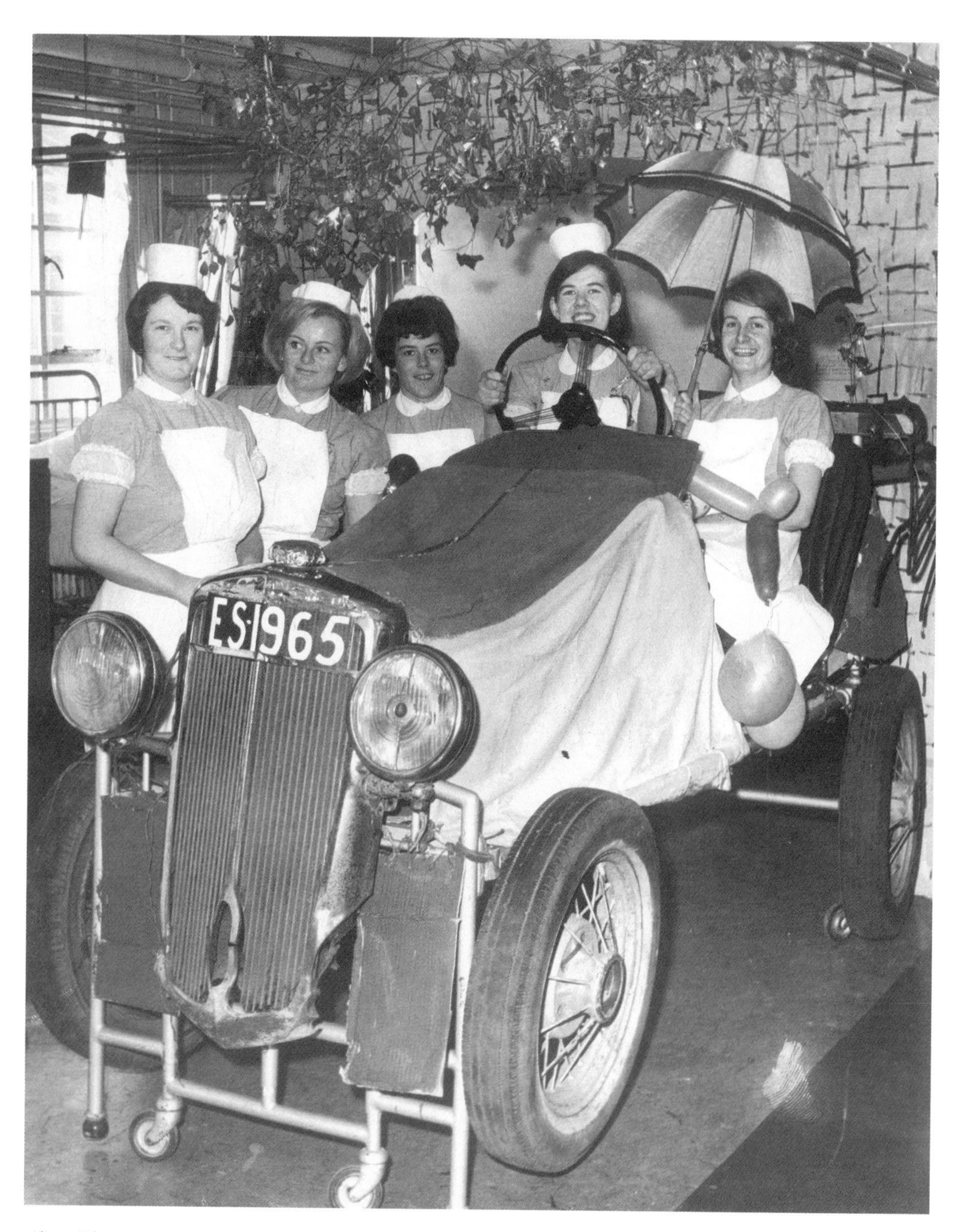

Above: These nurses on Bevers ward created some Christmas entertainment in 1965 by declaring one end of the ward Hyde Park and the other the Brighton seafront and creating the Bevers Special 'Bedstead flyer' jalopy to make the journey between them. (*Oxford Mail and Times*)

Opposite above: In 1973 Father Christmas cheered the day for Natasha Gavin, twenty-two months, a patient on Leopold ward. Sister June Hutt and Noddy joined in the fun. (*Oxford Mail and Times*)

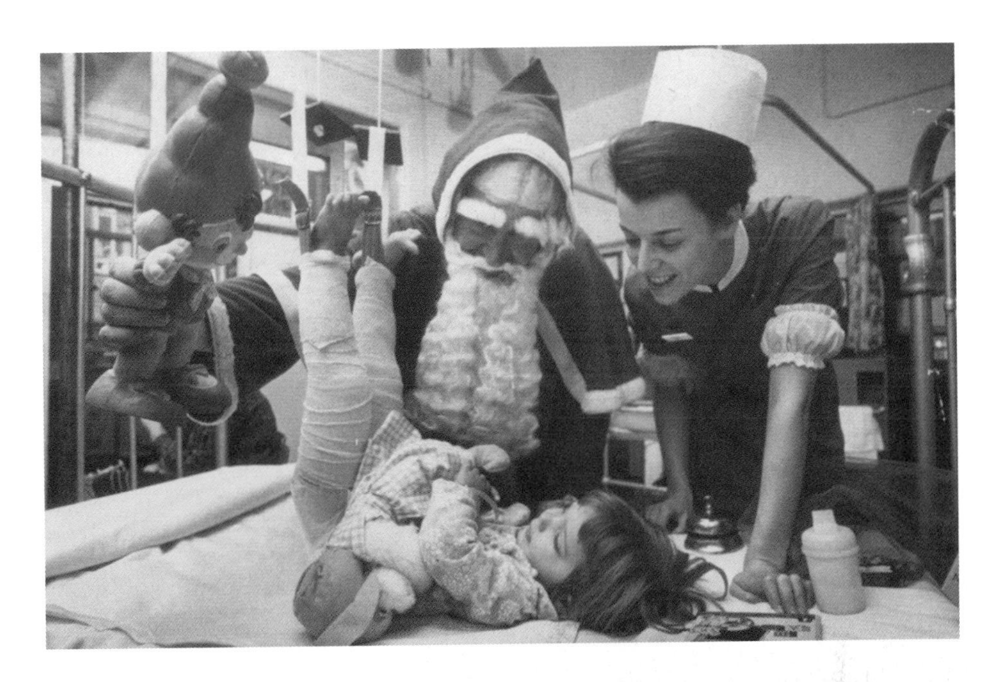

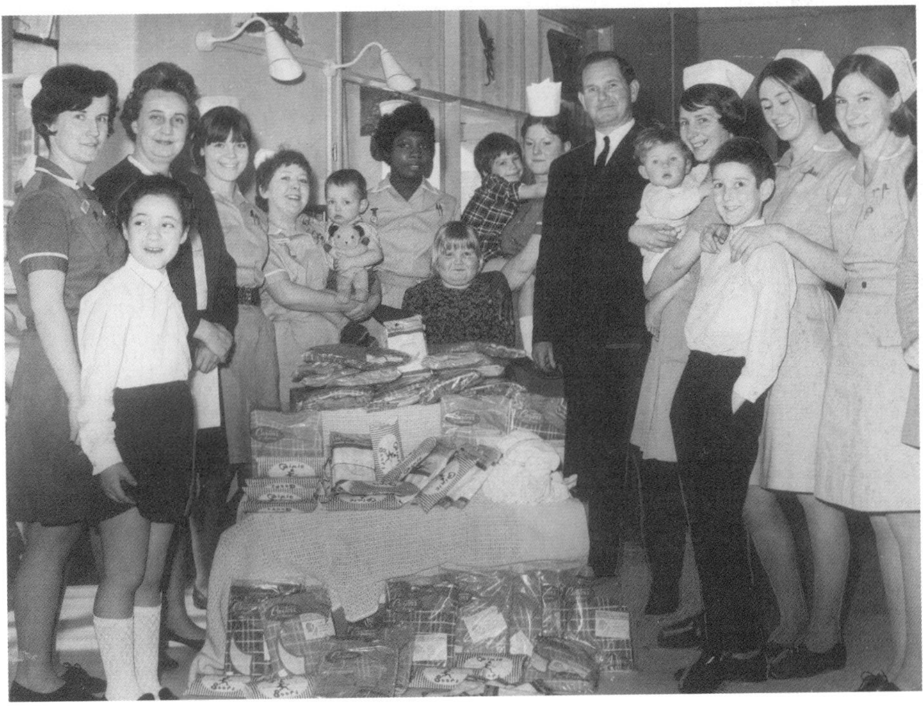

Oxford Rugby Football Club chose the Radcliffe Infirmary to receive some of the proceeds from a sports gala at its southern by-pass ground in 1970. Club players were often treated for injuries at the Infirmary, so as a thank you, the club – with help from Elliston and Cavell's department store (now Debenhams) – presented the four children's wards with a selection of clothes. Club chairman Eric Church is seen handing over the gifts in Leopold ward to Miss J. Mair, senior nursing officer (second left). (*Oxford Mail and Times*)

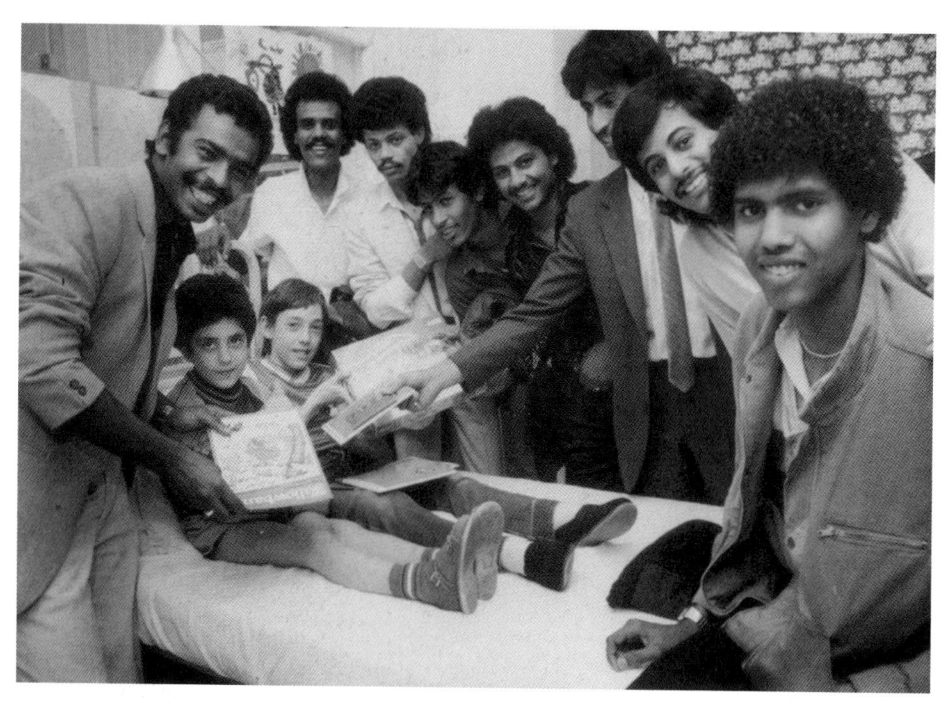

Students from Saudi Arabia studying at Oxford Academy brought a smile to the faces of children in hospital in 1975 when they marked the start of Ramadan with gifts of pens, bricks and toys. (*Oxford Mail and Times*)

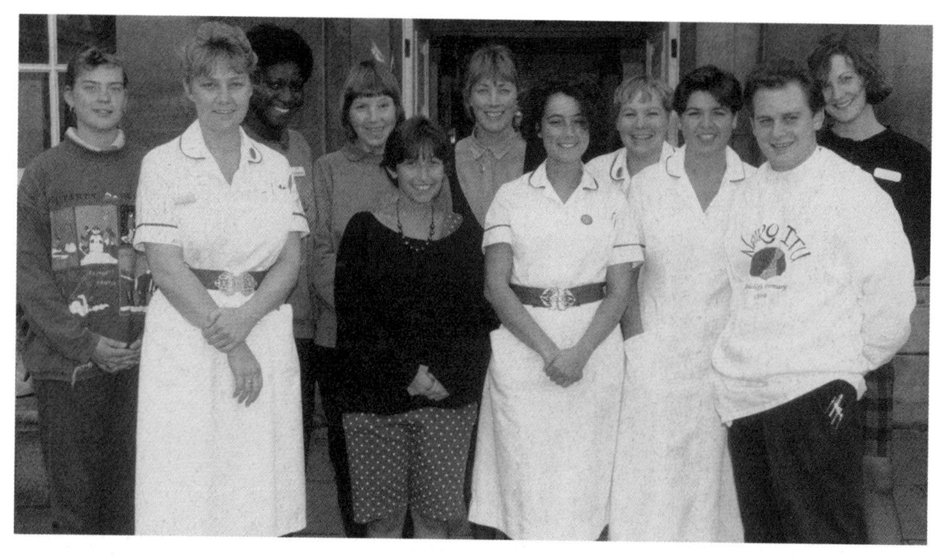

This cheery group of staff from Geoffrey Harris, Sherrington and Towler wards took part in a sponsored dash over a naval assault course near Bath in 1992 to raise money for the neurology department. They finished exhausted and covered in mud but raised £2,000. Nurse Mandy Collins (front left) organised the trip and top fundraiser was Jenny Dowdeswell (fourth from right), ward clerk on Sherrington. Judy Withers, now Matron for Neurosciences, is third from left. (*Oxford Mail and Times*)

Right: Images from the 'Tynchwycke' pantomime, *c.* 1960. The idea of the Christmas pantomime began in 1938 when the matron, Margaret Bonthron, asked the doctors to put on something for the second part of the nurses' concert. In 1940 it became *Dick Whittington and his Dog*, then came *Babes in the Ward* and a gradual change to the tradition of amusing ridicule of personalities and departments. Later titles included *Look back in Rigor*, *Handsome and Dettol* and *Lady Chatterley's Liver*. The name comes from Nicholas Tynchwycke who was the first known medical teacher at the university, a Fellow of Balliol and physician to Edward I.

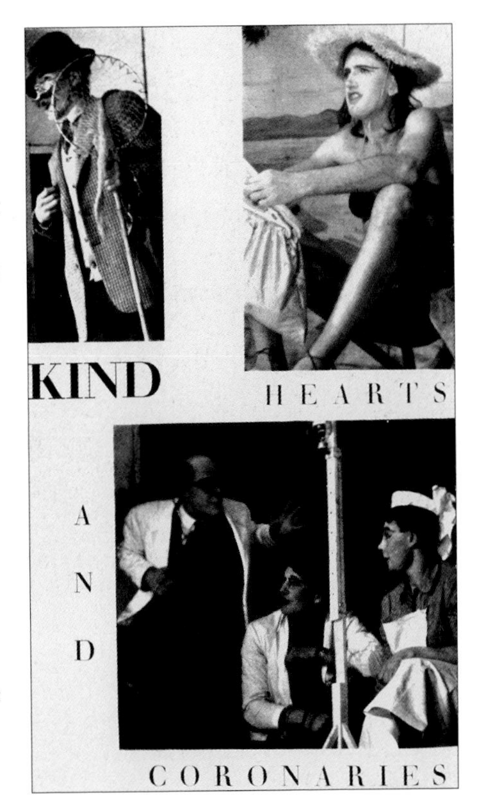

Below: An almoner interviews a patient, *c.* 1959. Almoners were on-the-spot social workers. Trained in psychology and social science, they provided practical and emotional support to people with worries and problems brought about or made worse by their hospital stay. Future almoners often did their part of their training at the Infirmary.

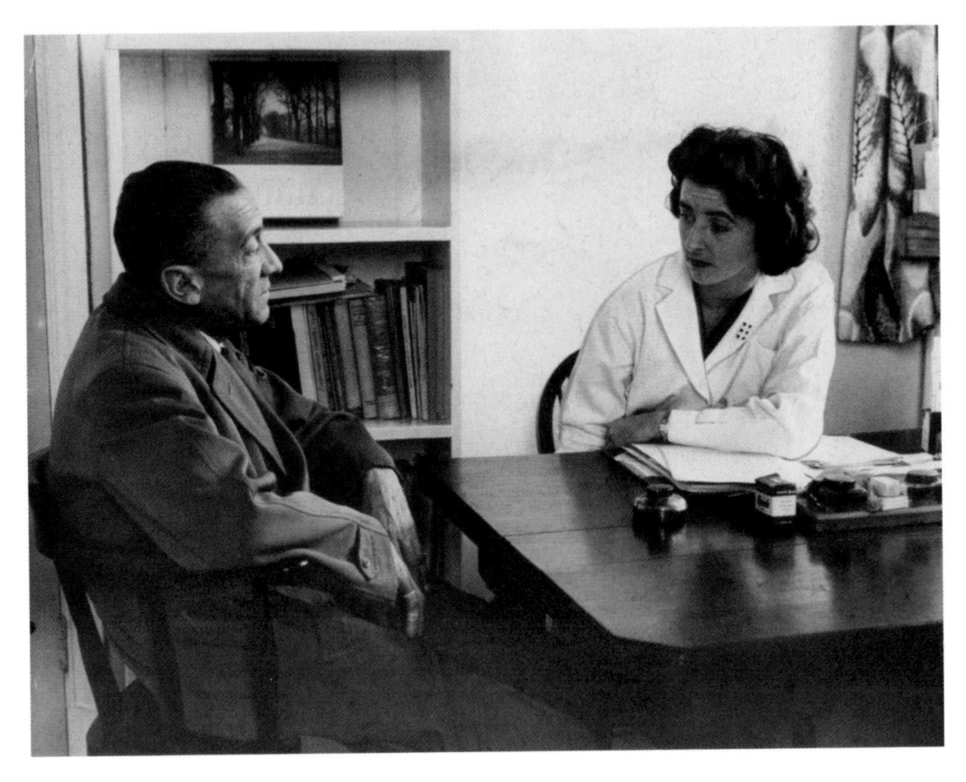

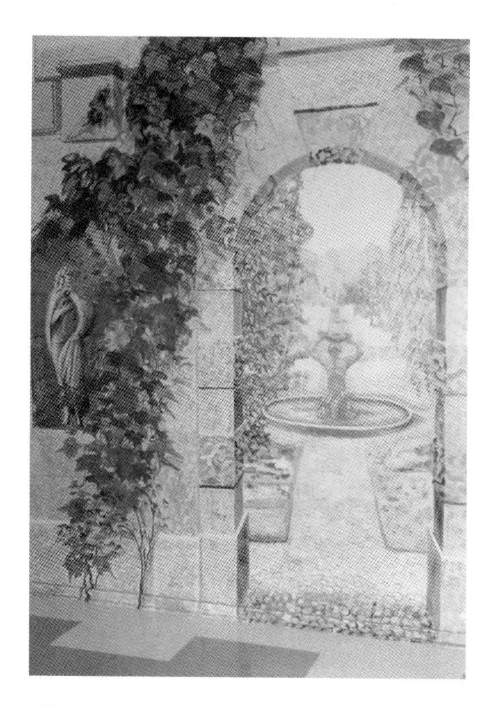

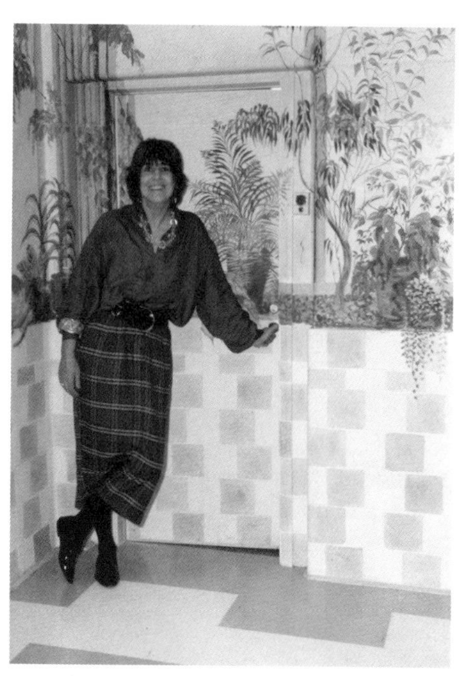

Above left and right: Hospital art. In the 1980s hospitals began to be more imaginative in the use of art as therapy for anxious patients. One of the most successful was the transformation of the,'cold, draughty and windowless' X-ray waiting room where artist Sarah Tisdall created an airy conservatory with shrubs and flowers and blue sky. The work brought new life to a dull area. (*Oxford Mail and Times*)

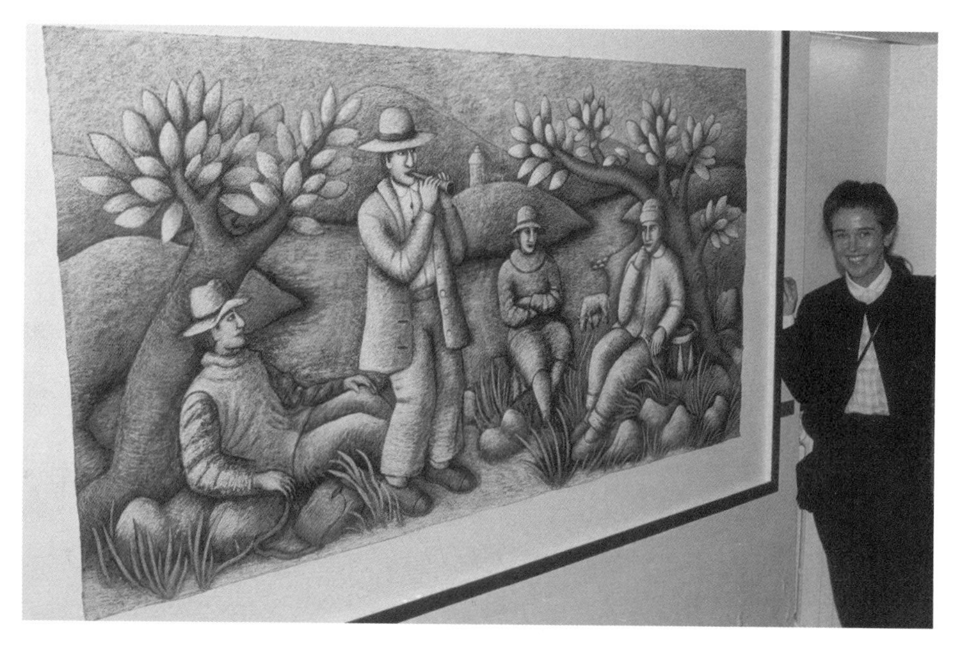

Artist Suzanne Driscoll, from Bicester, painted a landscape and an interior scene in her characteristic style for the front entrance. (*Oxford Mail and Times*)

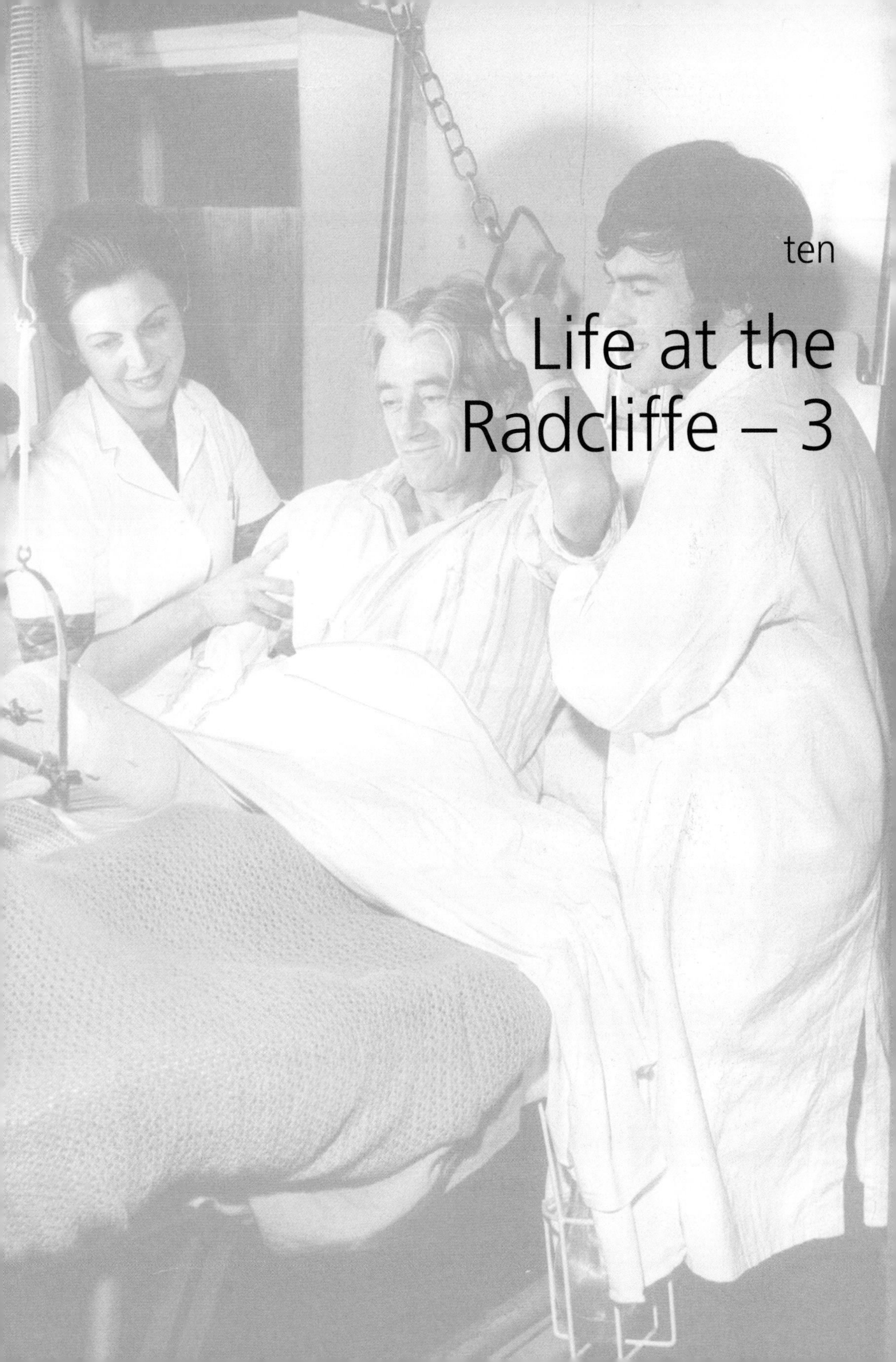

ten

Life at the Radcliffe – 3

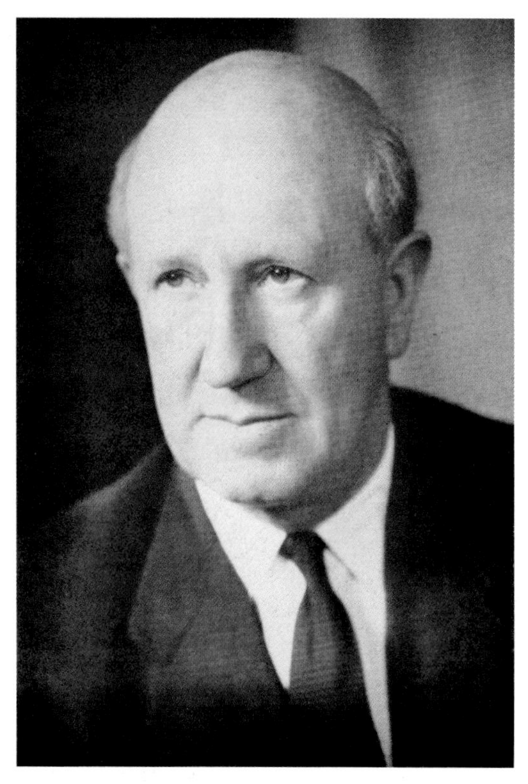

Dr Alec Cooke was the first consultant physician to be appointed in 1933 (until then physicians had all been in general practice as well). He had a special interest in metabolic disorders and founded a diabetic clinic in 1941. A man of wide ranging interests, he was famed for observations which became 'Cooke's laws' which included: 'It always takes longer than you think,' 'It costs more than you think' and 'A minor operation is always done on somebody else.'

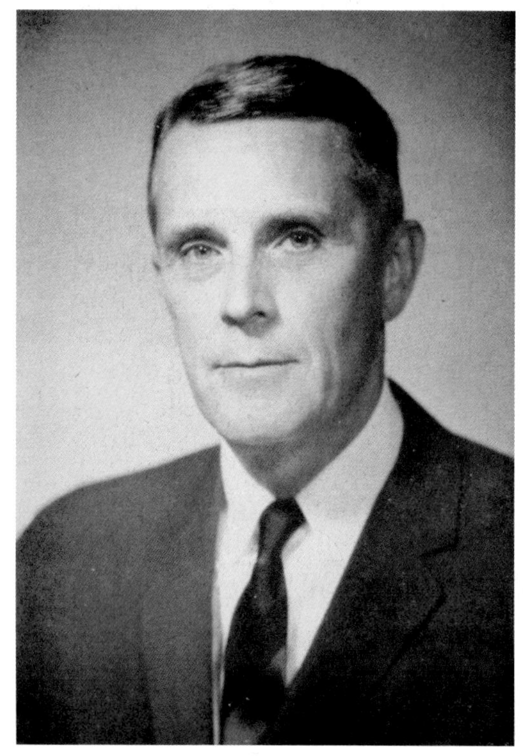

Professor Paul Beeson. It was a measure of the standing of the Radcliffe Infirmary that it was able to attract Paul Beeson, the physician in chief and chairman of the Department of Medicine at Yale University to become Nuffield Professor of Clinical Medicine at Oxford in 1965. He was a stimulating teacher, skilled scientist, able administrator and wise physician, highly regarded for his warm and friendly manner matched with a firm and decisive approach.

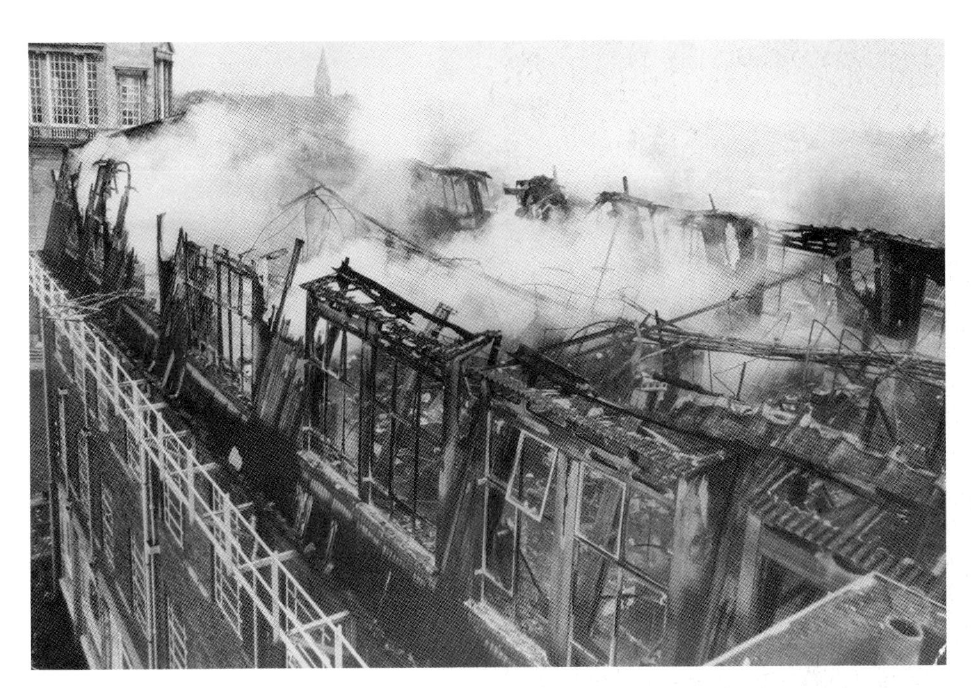

Fire disaster

In March 1971 a disastrous fire destroyed the medical library and offices on the top floor of Nuffield wing. More than 120 patients from the wards below were evacuated – including four from the intensive care unit immediately below the fire. One was kept alive by artificial respiration during the move.

The alarm was raised just after 3 a.m. In all, seven wards were evacuated, with some patients able to walk and others being carried by nurses, doctors, porters, police and medical students. Charred paper and blackened rubble were all that remained of the precious collections of books and papers in the Cairns library. (*Oxford Mail and Times*)

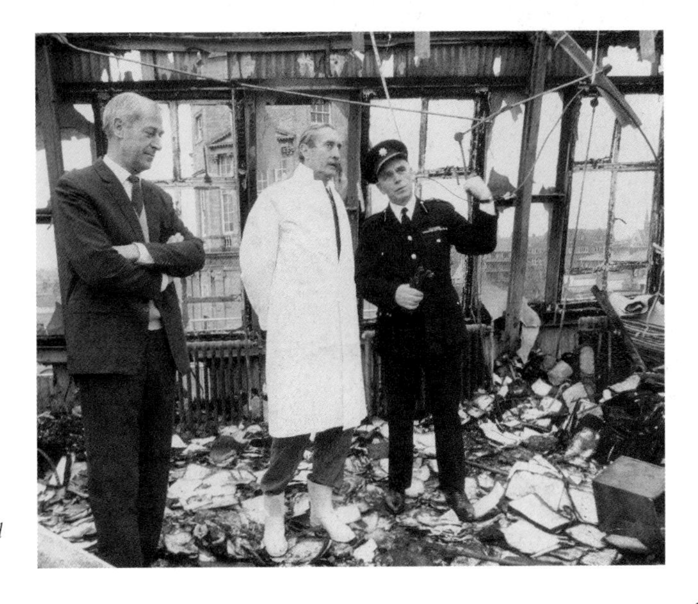

Chief officer of Oxford City Fire Brigade, Mr Sidney Boulter, showing the damage to the Lord Mayor, Alderman Michael Maclagan (in white coat) and John Spencer, administrator of United Oxford Hospitals. John Spencer was later administrator for Oxfordshire Area Health Authority. (*Oxford Mail and Times*)

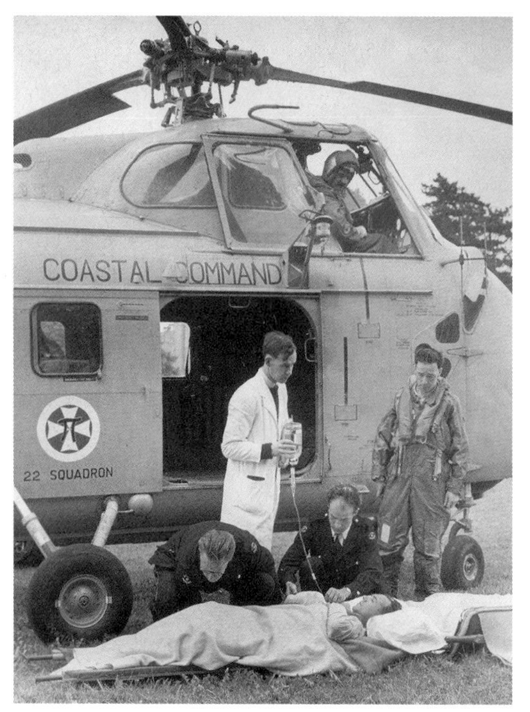

Left and below: Helicopter landings Patients from all over the country were frequently flown to the Infirmary because of its specialist skills. Usually, the helicopters landed in the university parks.

These pictures show a man being treated after a flight from Barnstaple in Devon (1960) and an eight-year-old boy from Liverpool who was the first patient to be flown in by night in 1962. The landing was at the Pressed Steel (now BMW) sports ground. The ambulance, fire engine, police cars and private cars shone their headlights onto a large canvas H and, as the helicopter approached, police lit flares to guide the pilot. (*Oxford Mail and Times*)

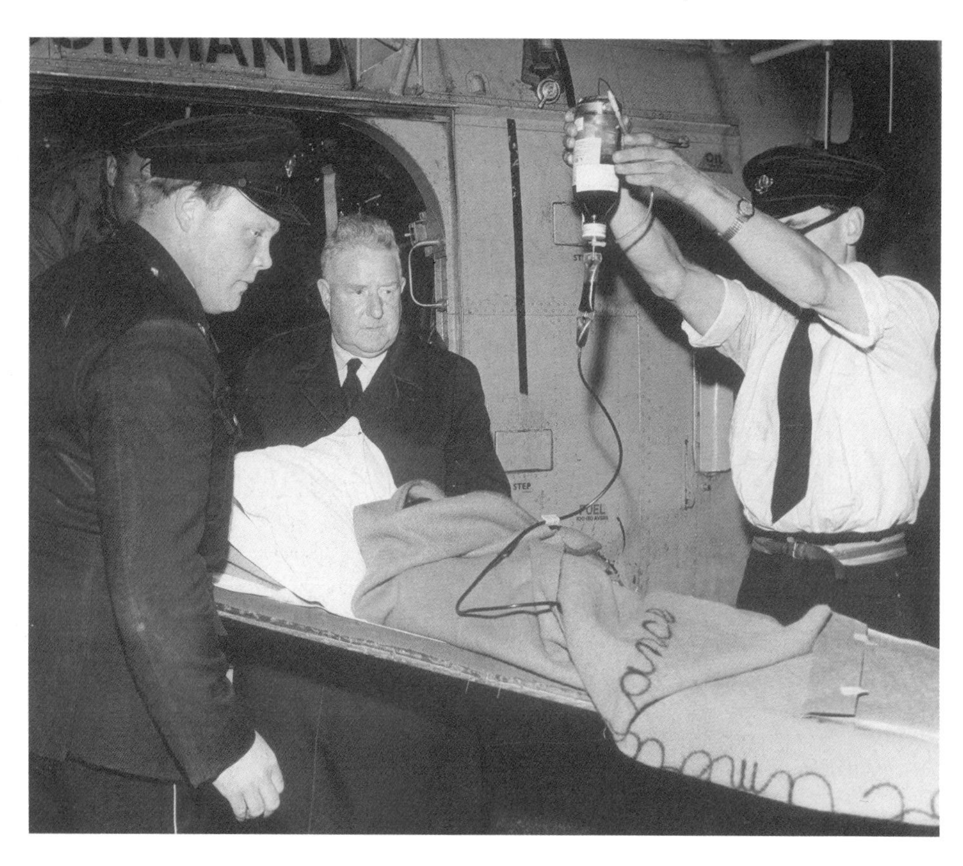

Right: David Wilson, appointed house governor in 1978. A popular and able manager, he successfully piloted the Infirmary through a period of change, becoming general manager in the 1980s, at a time when it was popular to appoint captains of industry to NHS posts, and chief executive when the hospital became an NHS Trust in the 1990s. He left in 1997 to become chief executive of Northampton General Hospital. (*Oxford Mail and Times*)

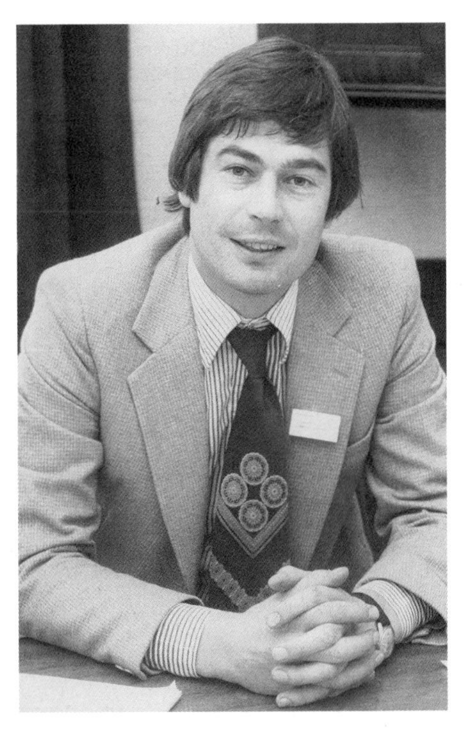

Below: Arthur Elliott-Smith casts a nostalgic glance behind him as he leaves in style on his retirement. He arrived in 1938, and apart from war service (when he rose to the rank of Brigadier) he was, 'one of the surgical cornerstones' of the hospital for over thirty years. A master craftsman, he made all his operations appear easy and created a happy atmosphere in the theatre.

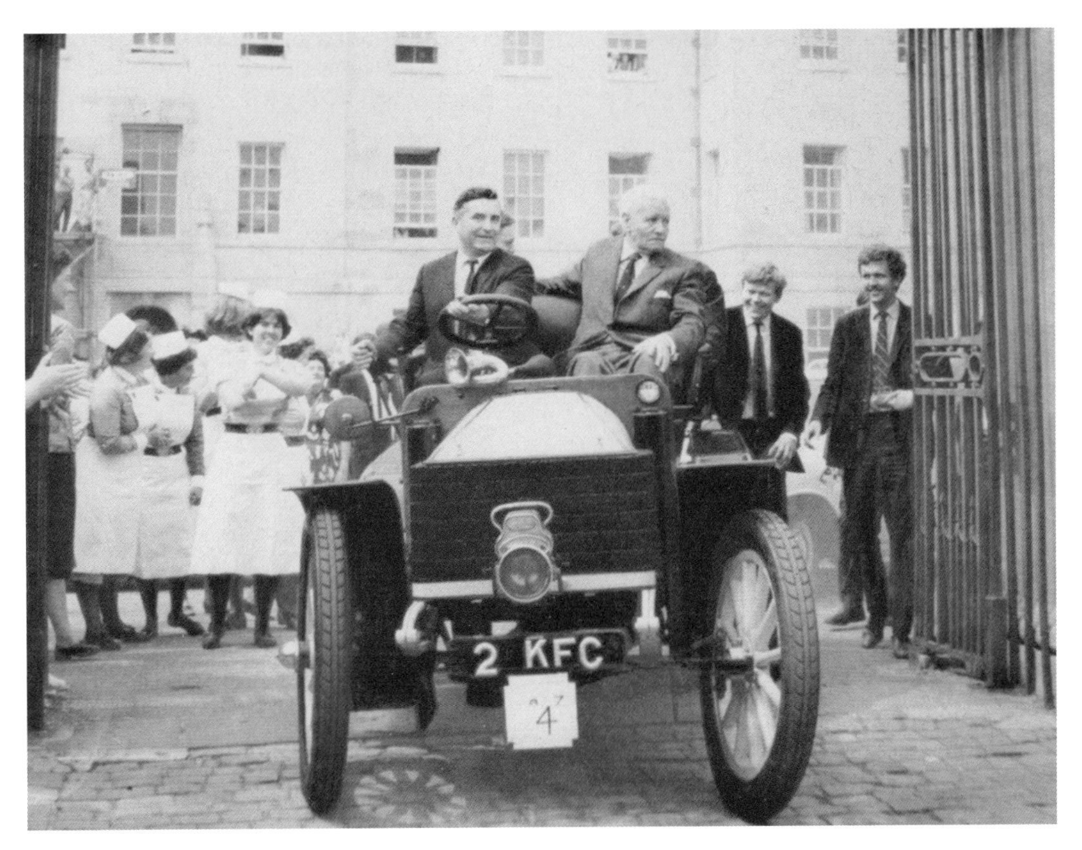

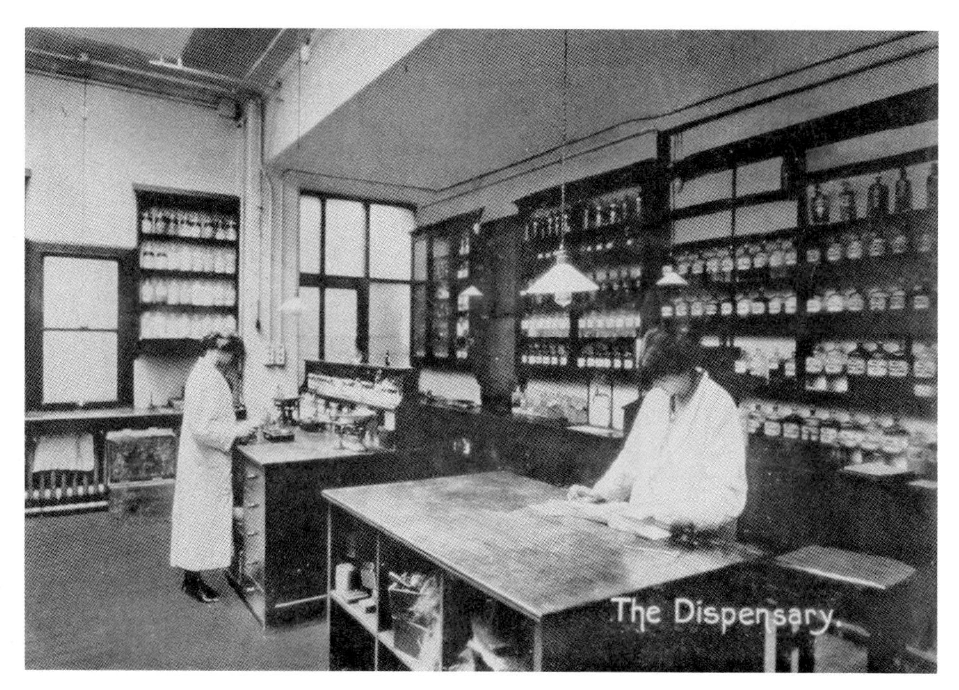

Pharmacy

The pharmacy dispensary, *c.* 1922.

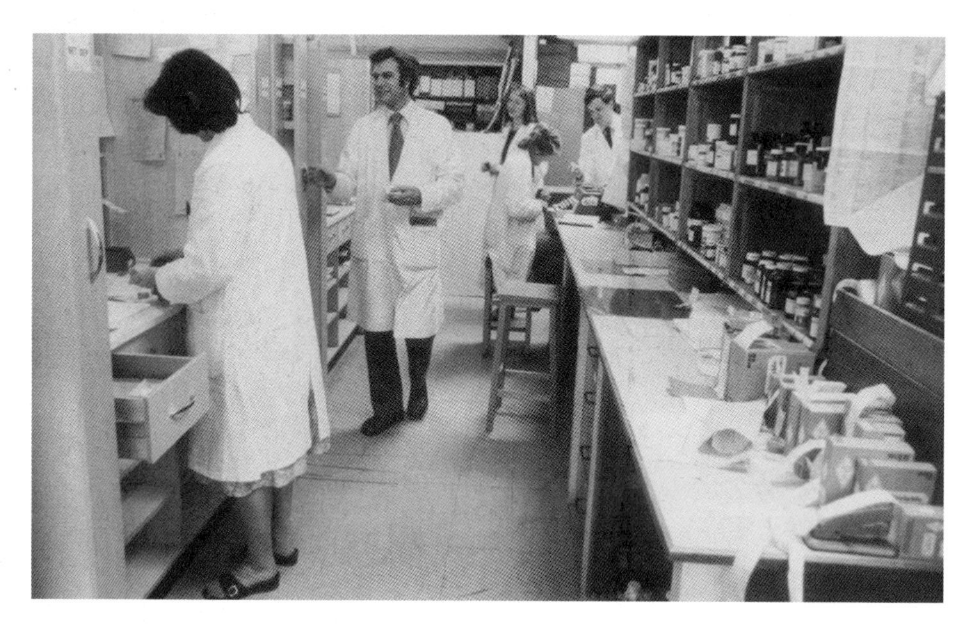

The hospital had a long history of making its own drugs and medicines but in 1978 a report by the medicines inspector described conditions in the pharmacy as 'exceedingly cramped, poorly equipped, furnished and decorated and a most unsuitable environment for the manufacture of medicinal products'. Similar criticisms were applied to other Oxford hospitals and before long such work was concentrated at the Churchill Hospital. (*Oxford Mail and Times*)

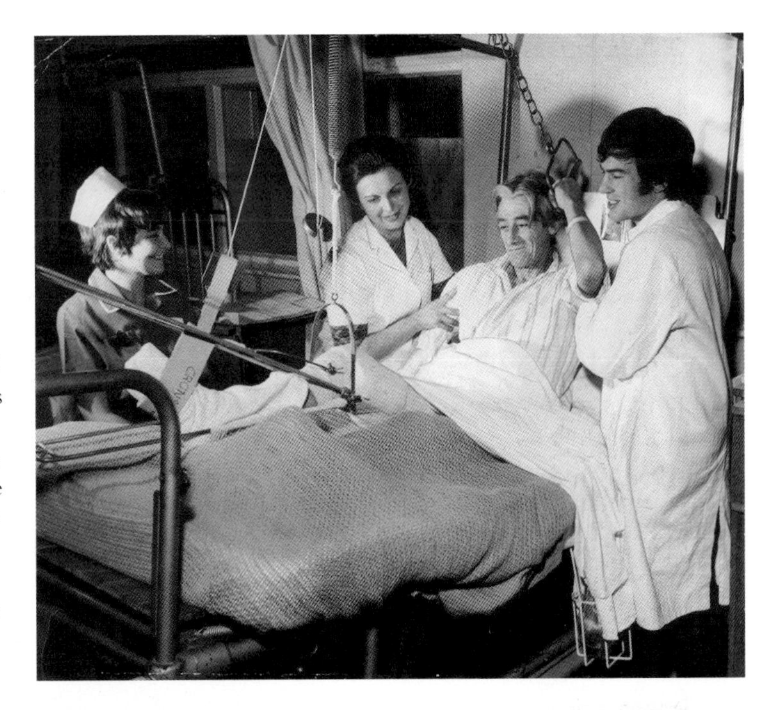

So serious was the flu outbreak in early 1970 that the hospital appealed for volunteers to help staff the wards. The public responded eagerly and both trained and untrained volunteers played their part on the wards or in non-nursing departments. The picture shows a medical student and a volunteer helping out during the crisis. A similar crisis occurred in 1973. (*Oxford Mail and Times*)

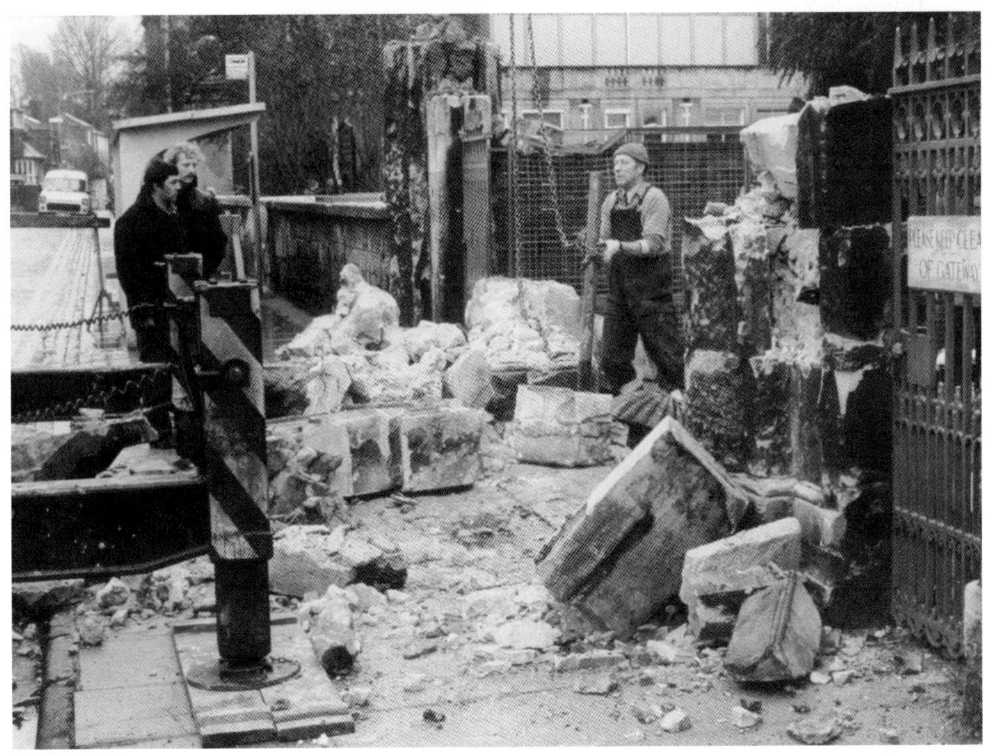

The pillars at the front gate suffered one knock too many in 1977 when a heavy vehicle crashed into them and left them unstable. They had to be demolished but were replaced by a new set on the same site as 200 years before.

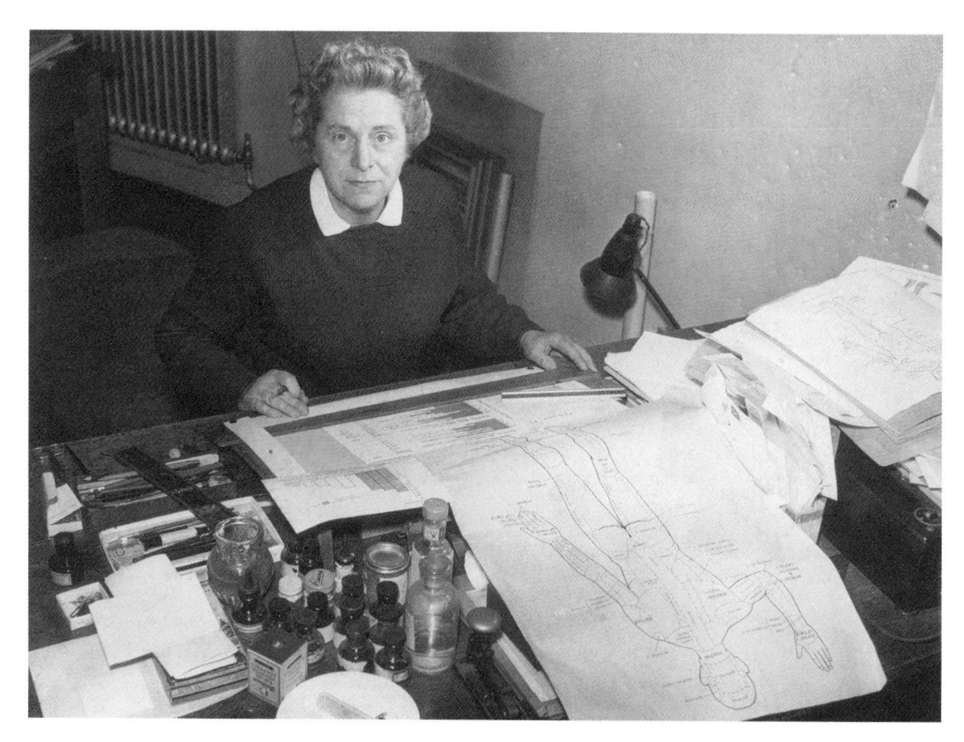

Above and below: In the days before digital images, powerpoint, DVD and videotape the task of recording images for clinical records and for teaching material was done by artists drawing freehand and photographers working with black and white film. These pictures from 1959 show Margaret McLarty working on an illustration for a medical text book and photographer Eric Tugwell taking a picture of a baby's hand. (*Oxford Mail and Times*)

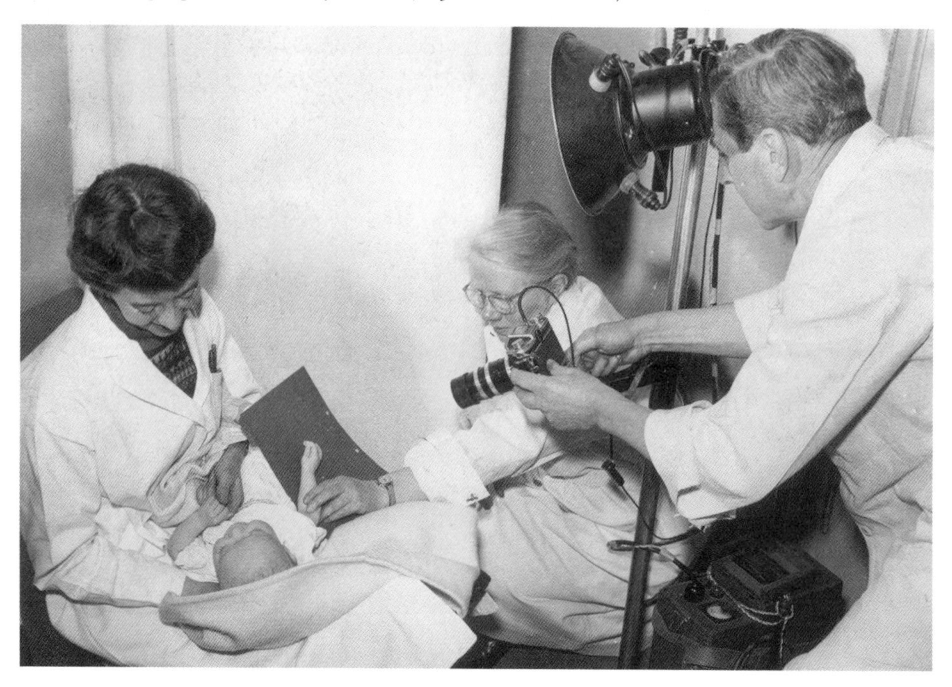

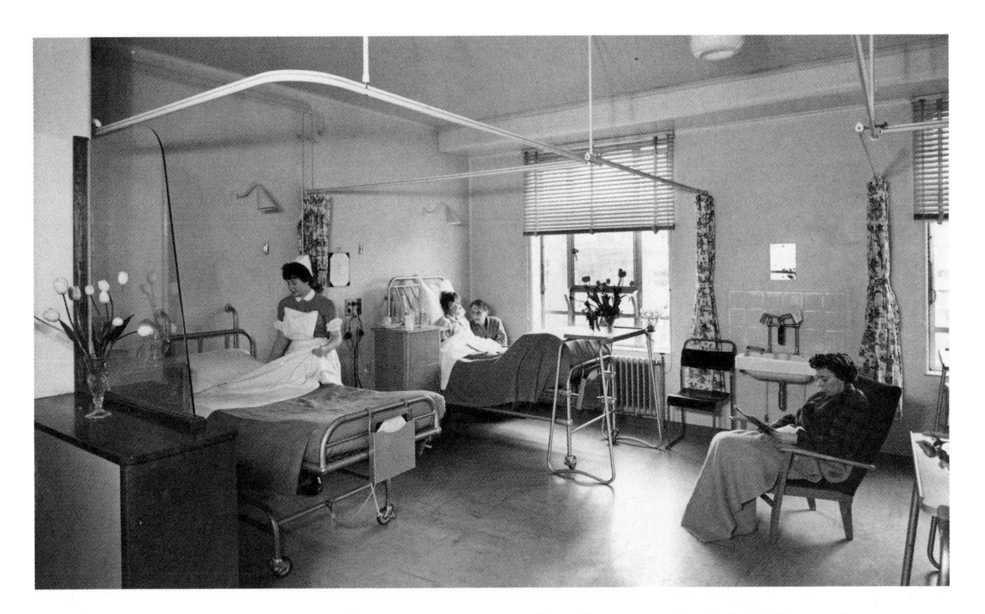

In 1958 the new wards in the Nuffield Department of Medicine received their first patients. Before they opened, Professor Witts proudly showed them to a party of guests and told them, 'We think these may be the finest hospital wards in the country.'

He pledged that the department would take its full share of the work of the hospital and, 'maintain the close relationship with the city which is such a special feature of the Radcliffe'.

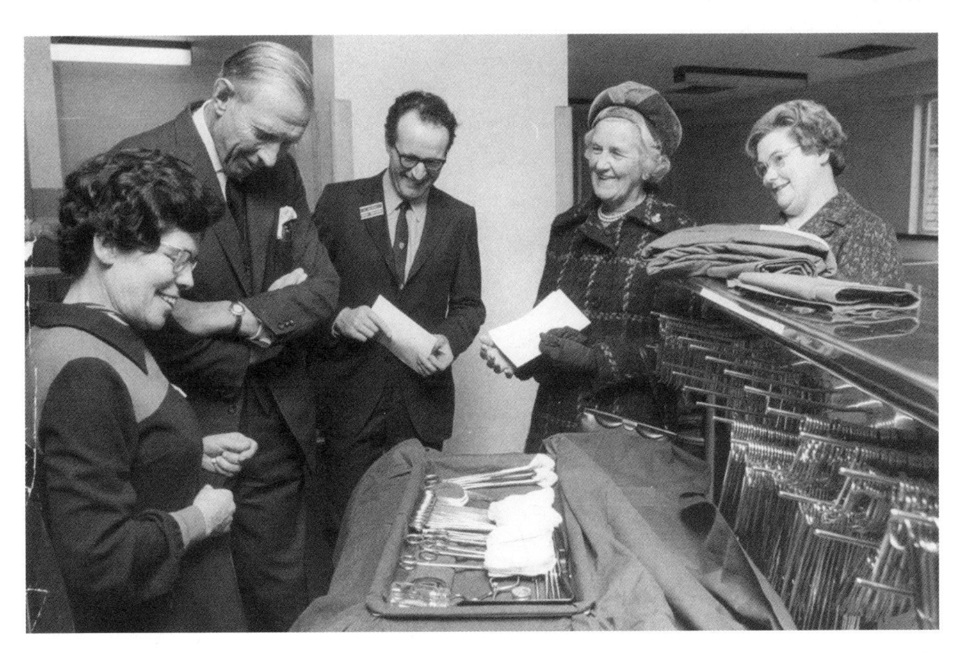

Col. Sir John Thomson, Lord-Lieutenant of Oxfordshire, opened the £542,000 Towler Block in 1972, which included four new theatres and an eight-bed intensive therapy unit. It was completed less than a decade before the John Radcliffe Hospital opened, thanks to the persistence of the United Oxford Hospitals chairman Eric Towler, who made it clear to the Department of Health that patching up and making do was not good enough.

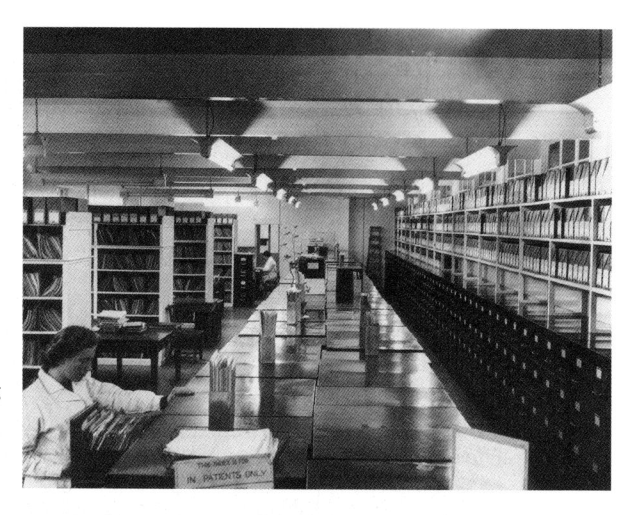

Right: A crisis in medical records: in the 1950s the medical records were entirely on paper and stored in row upon row of shelving. Staff wore white coats (so that it was clear to patients and visitors who they were) and also dealt with registering patients, booking appointments and organising waiting lists. A statistician worked in a separate office, providing returns for the Ministry of Health. (*Oxford Mail and Times*)

Records were growing at the rate of a metre a day in the 1970s, with half a million stored in the basement of the Infirmary. In the 1960s the department could store 100 records in a foot of shelving, but record-keeping grew more detailed and the files so thick that there was now only room for twenty-five. Microfilming had been tried, but was expensive and not very user friendly. It was proving a real headache for managers.

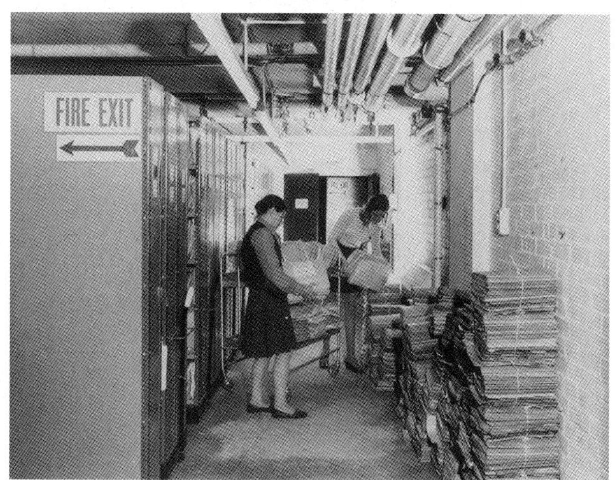

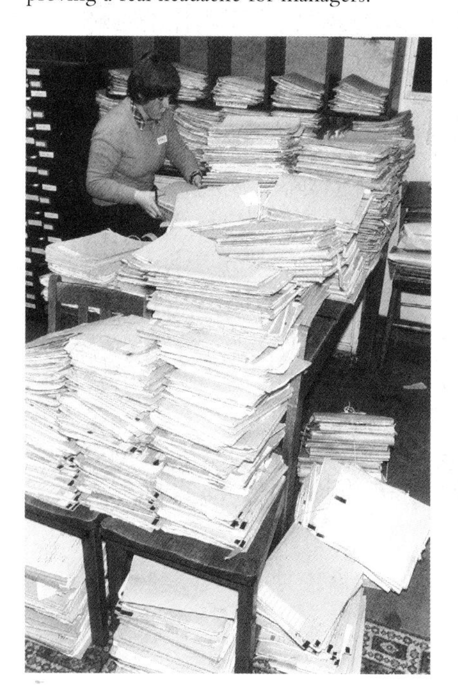

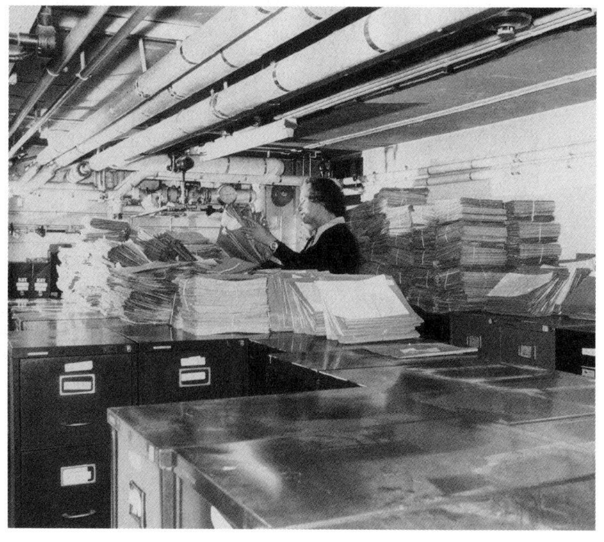

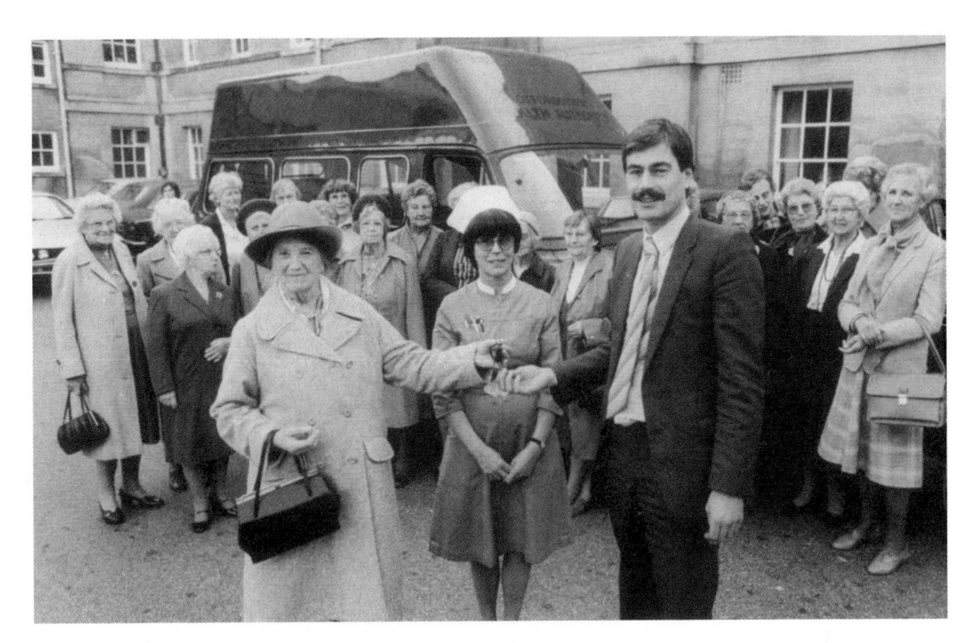

Volunteers who had sold refreshments in outpatients since the 1930s ended their service in 1983 when the League of Friends took over their role. They used their remaining funds to buy a £9,300 minibus which they handed to general manager David Wilson. (*Oxford Mail and Times*)

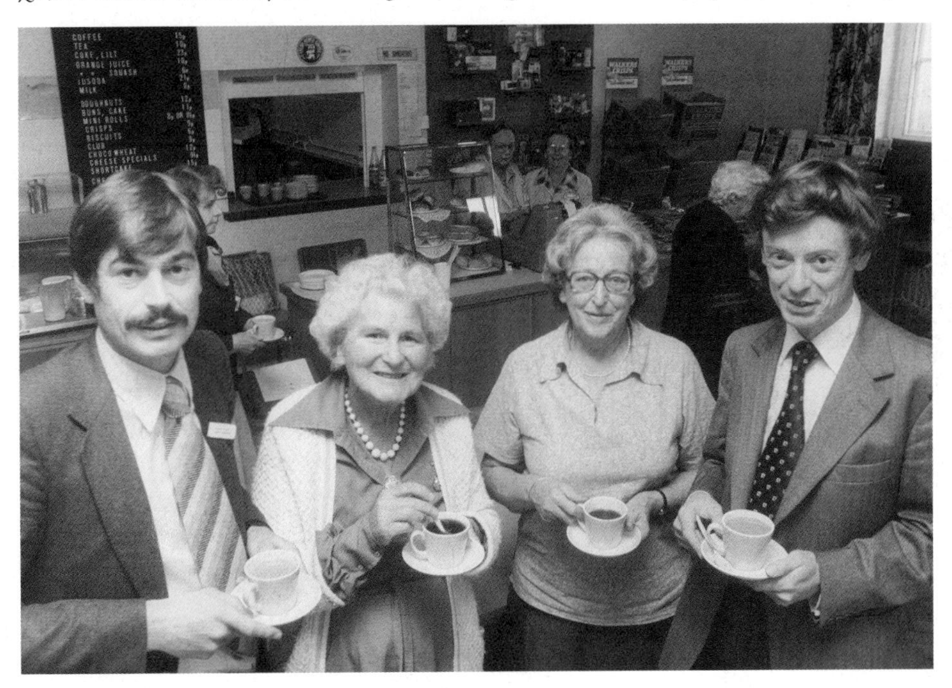

The official opening of the new League of Friends cafeteria in 1981. With David Wilson are Lady Radcliffe-Maud (president of the League) Mrs Mary Bird (chairman) and Charles Moorley (treasurer). At the time tea was 10p and coffee 15p. The popular cafeteria provided a much-valued service to patients, visitors and staff over many years and contributed thousands of pounds to hospital funds. (*Oxford Mail and Times*)

Two men who were to feature prominently in Oxford heart medicine in the next thirty years are in this picture from 1970, receiving a cheque for £6,000 for equipment to help in blood pressure studies. Dr Peter Sleight, consultant physician (centre) and Dr Brian Gribbin, research fellow, are seen here with Michael Rowntree (extreme right) who was chairman of the finance committee of the Board of Governors, and Brigadier E. Cardiff, director general of the British Heart Foundation. (*Oxford Mail and Times*)

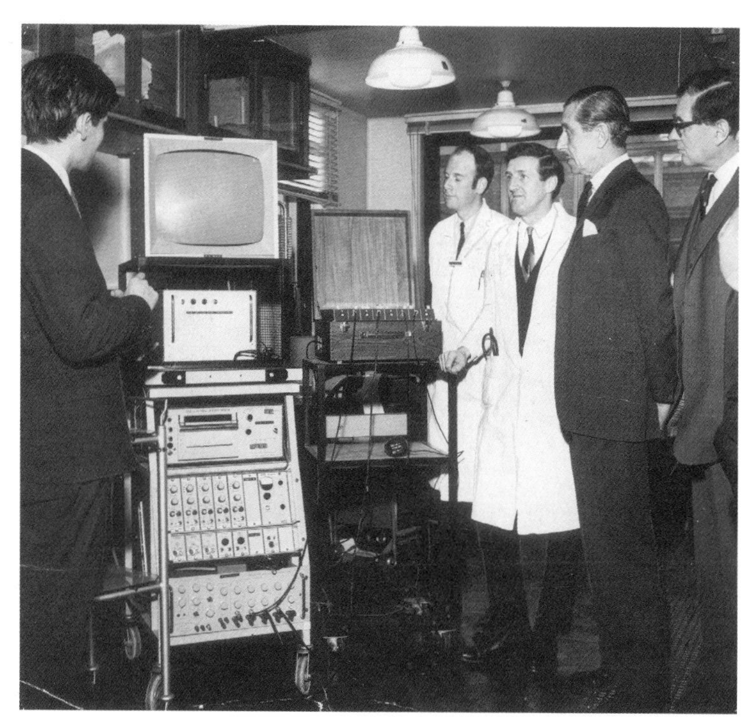

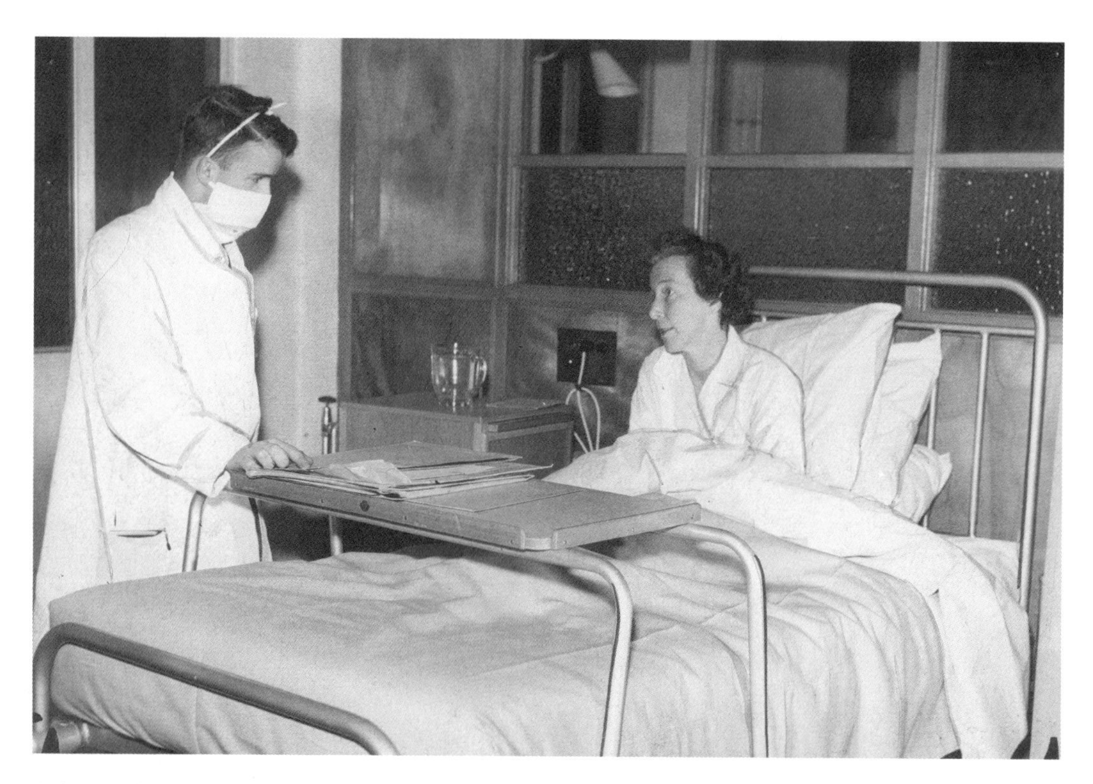

A doctor talks to the first patient in the new Nuffield Department of Surgery which opened in 1958. The department included wards, an operating theatre and facilities for research and teaching.

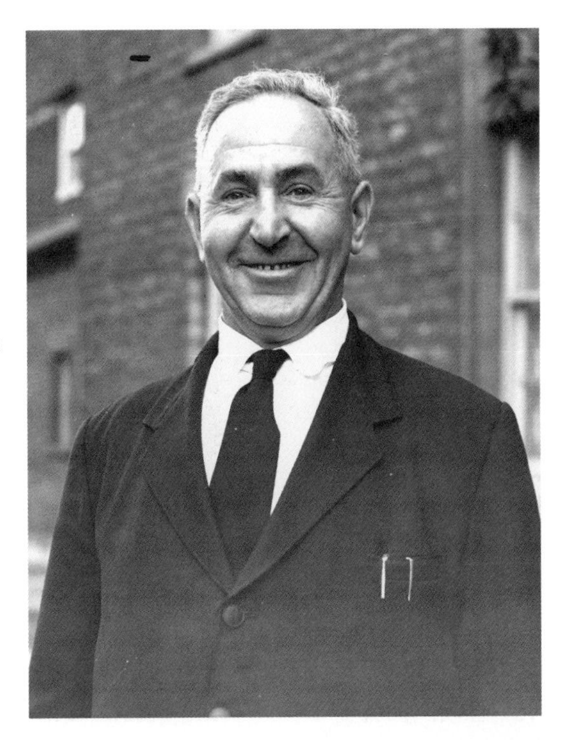

Right: William Woodward who retired as head porter in 1958 after thirty-seven years. He recalled working fifteen hours a day on occasions and never had a complete Christmas at home. (Oxfordshire County Council Photographic Archives – Newsquest)

Below: Kenneth White, pathology technician, celebrated forty years at the hospital in 1970 by raising a glass with Alastair Robb-Smith. His father had been on the maintenance staff of the engineer's department from 1920-36 and his uncle, William Woodward, was head porter. His son Nick was later a hospital photographer. (Oxfordshire County Council Photographic Archives – Newsquest)

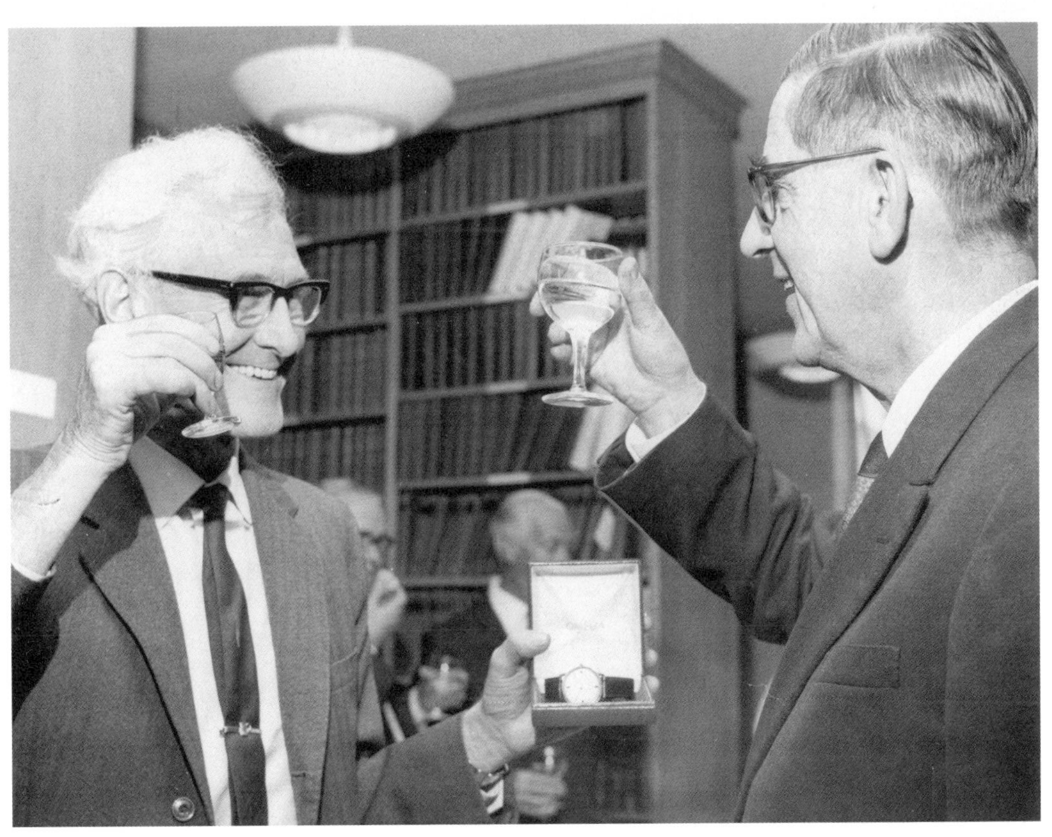

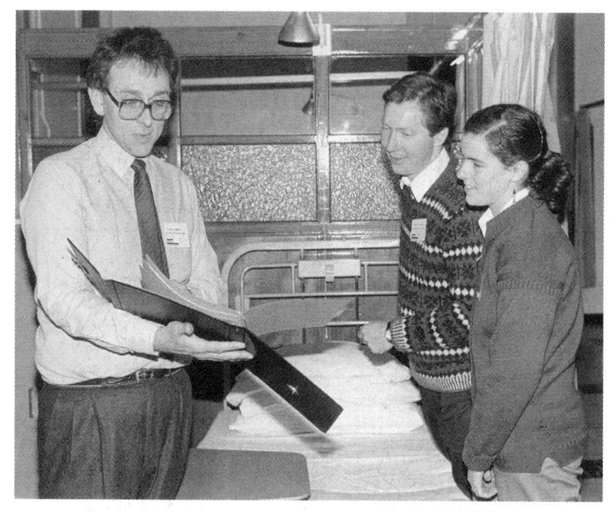

Senior nurse Alan Pearson with nurse practitioners Kate Atkinson and Richard McMahon on Beeson ward which became a Nursing Development Unit in the mid-1980s, introducing a new and more informal style of care for rehabilitation patients. The unit attracted national attention and was visited by many nurses who introduced similar methods in their own hospitals. (*Oxford Mail and Times*)

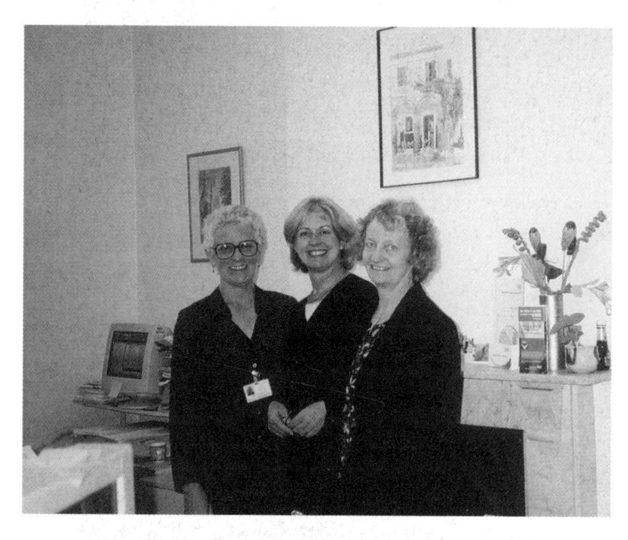

Three of the many unsung heroines who have served the Radcliffe Infirmary with dedication and commitment. Valerie Thompson, Kathy Gardner and Brenda Spiess worked together in administration for most of the last two decades.

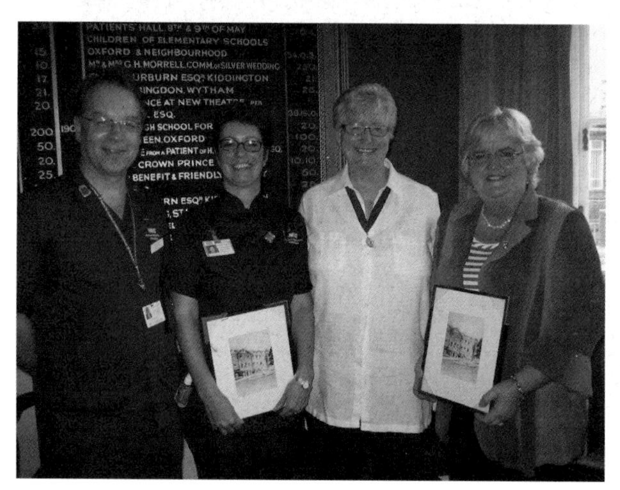

The achievements of nursing at the RI were remembered when the Chief Nursing Officer for England, Chris Beasley (right), visited the hospital in July 2006. With her, from left to right, are: Steve Candler, Associate Chief Nurse, Division B (the most senior nurse at the RI), Julie Hartley-Jones, former Director of Nursing at the RI and later Chief Nurse for Oxford Radcliffe Hospitals and Sue Buckingham, President of the Radcliffe Infirmary Guild of Nurses.

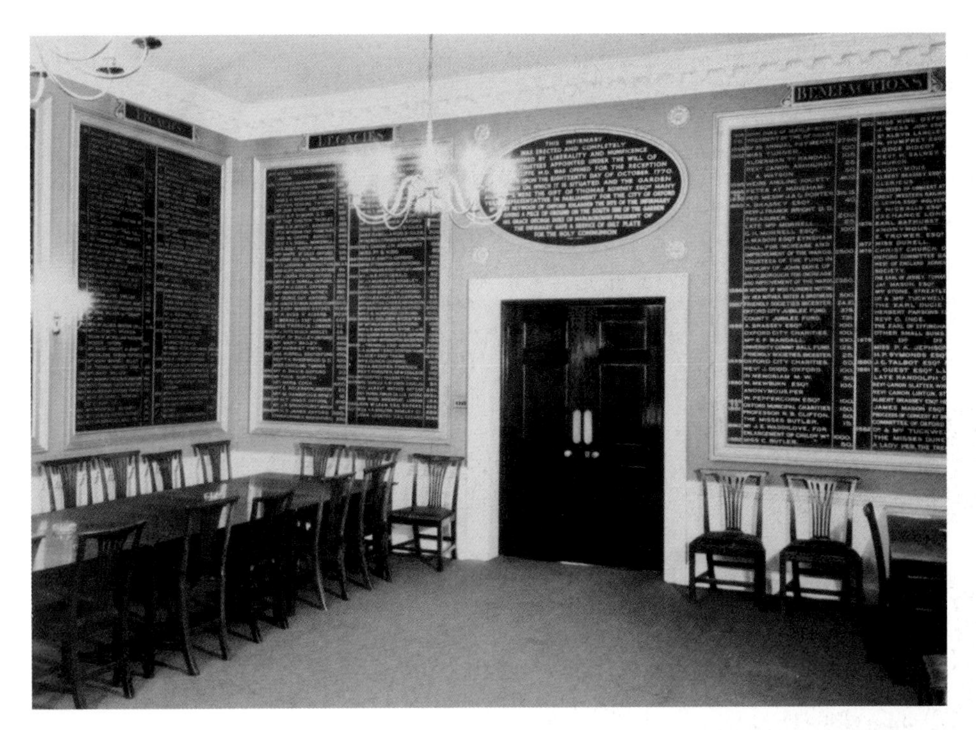

Above and below: The board room and the plaque which records the generosity of the original founders, photographed in 1975. The room and its chairs are unchanged in over 200 years, a symbol of continuity in a hospital which has seen momentous achievements and vast change. Clinical services have now moved to modern buildings at Headington to join the mainstream of Oxford's hospital services. The eighteenth-century building now starts a new era with Oxford University.

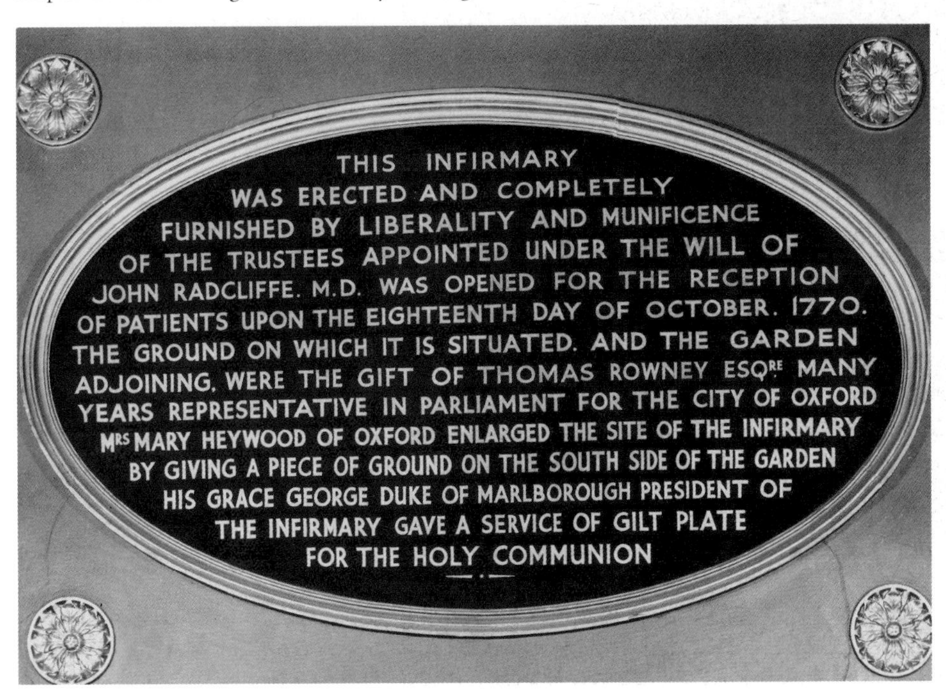

Other local titles published by Tempus

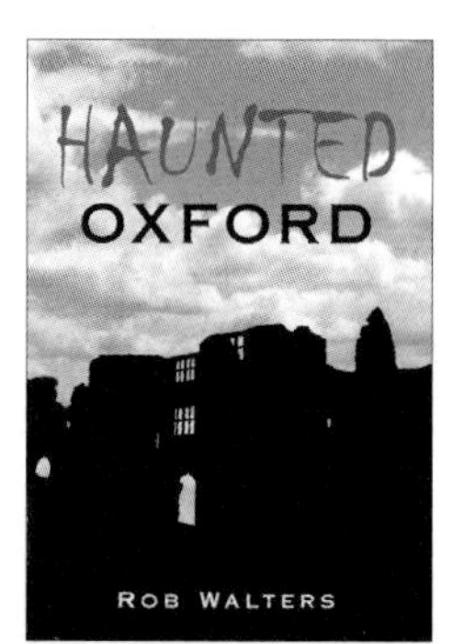

Haunted Oxford

ROB WALTERS

From heart-stopping accounts of apparitions, manifestations and related supernatural phenomena to first-hand encounters with ghouls and spirits, this collection of stories contains new and well-known spooky tales from around the historic city of Oxford. From tales of spirits that haunt the libraries of the Oxford Colleges to stories of spectral monks and even royal ghosts, this gathering of ghostly goings-on will captivate anyone interested in the supernatural history of the area.

0 7524 3925 1

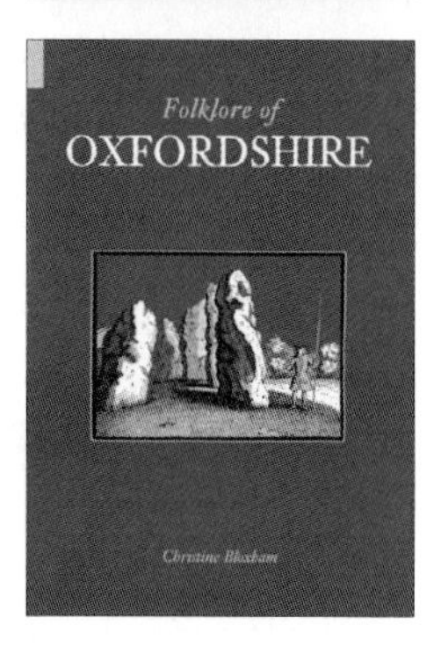

Folklore of Oxfordshire

CHRISTINE BLOXHAM

Oxfordshire's heritage is reflected in the diversity of its customs and folklore. Especially rich in traditions, dialect and vocabulary, legends and wondrous stories that have been handed down through the ages, the character of Oxfordshire and its people is firmly rooted in its folklore. *Folklore of Oxfordshire* contains many examples of these and more and will delight all those who wish to revel in the delights of times past.

0 7524 3664 3

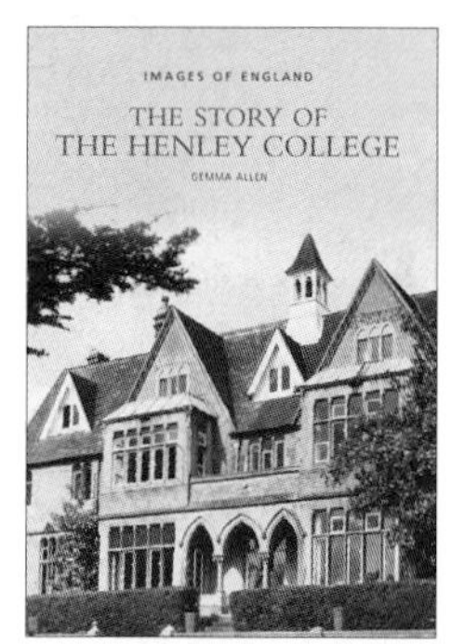

The Story of the Henley College

GEMMA ALLEN

In this fascinating collection of photographs, engravings and prints the origins of The Henley College are told. Readers will discover how changes in the education system and the fortunes of local benefactors transformed the college from the seventeenth-century Free Grammar School, into the eighteenth-century United Charities School, which in turn became the Henley Grammar School in the run up to the First World War, and in 1987 The Henley College as it is known today.

0 7524 3246 X

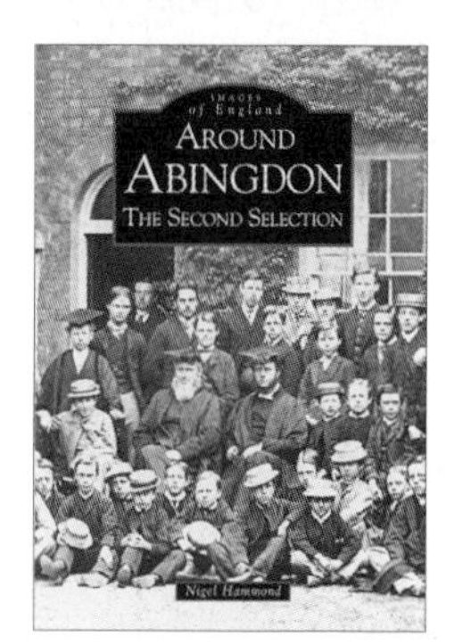

Around Abingdon The Second Selection

NIGEL HAMMOND

This second selection of photographs and illustrations of the Abingdon area recalls a bygone era that has seen dramatic changes over the years. In the eighteenth and nineteenth centuries Abingdon thrived as the county town of Berkshire, as an agricultural market and as a centre for manufacturing, commerce and trade. More recently, the MG car factory and the Atomic Energy Research Establishment at Harwell have led to its continued prosperity. The book will provide a nostalgic trip down memory lane.

0 7524 2649 4

If you are interested in purchasing other books published by Tempus, or in case you have difficulty finding any Tempus books in your local bookshop, you can also place orders directly through our website

www.tempus-publishing.com